IBS: Dietary advice to calm your gut

Alex Gazzola is a health journalist who has written for over 100 publications in 20 countries. He is the author of several other books, including *Living with Food Intolerance* and *Coeliac Disease: What you need to know*, both also published by Sheldon Press. He has a special interest in food allergies, digestive health and coeliac disease, about which he writes and blogs regularly. His website is at <www.alexgazzola.co.uk>.

Julie Thompson is a registered dietitian with a specialism in inflammatory and functional gut disorders and 'free from' diets for food intolerances and allergies. She is an adviser to the IBS Network, runs the Calm Gut Clinic (<www.calmgutclinic.co.uk>) in Yorkshire and works for the NHS part time. She is a regular contributor to *Network Health Dietitians* magazine, is a member of the UK BDA guideline development group for IBS and diet, and was a lay member on the NICE Quality Standards development for IBS.

Overcoming Common Problems Series

Selected titles

A full list of titles is available from Sheldon Press,
36 Causton Street, London SW1P 4ST and on our website at
www.sheldonpress.co.uk

Beating Insomnia: Without really trying
Dr Tim Cantopher

Birth Over 35
Sheila Kitzinger

Breast Cancer: Your treatment choices
Dr Terry Priestman

Chronic Fatigue Syndrome: What you need to know about CFS/ME
Dr Megan A. Arroll

The Chronic Pain Diet Book
Neville Shone

Cider Vinegar
Margaret Hills

Coeliac Disease: What you need to know
Alex Gazzola

Coping Successfully with Chronic Illness: Your healing plan
Neville Shone

Coping Successfully with Hiatus Hernia
Dr Tom Smith

Coping Successfully with Pain
Neville Shone

Coping Successfully with Panic Attacks
Shirley Trickett

Coping Successfully with Prostate Cancer
Dr Tom Smith

Coping Successfully with Shyness
Margaret Oakes, Professor Robert Bor and
Dr Carina Eriksen

Coping Successfully with Ulcerative Colitis
Peter Cartwright

Coping Successfully with Varicose Veins
Christine Craggs-Hinton

Coping Successfully with Your Irritable Bowel
Rosemary Nicol

Coping with a Mental Health Crisis: Seven steps to healing
Catherine G. Lucas

Coping with Anaemia
Dr Tom Smith

Coping with Asthma in Adults
Mark Greener

Coping with Blushing
Professor Robert J. Edelmann

Coping with Bronchitis and Emphysema
Dr Tom Smith

Coping with Chemotherapy
Dr Terry Priestman

Coping with Coeliac Disease: Strategies to change your diet and life
Karen Brody

Coping with Difficult Families
Dr Jane McGregor and Tim McGregor

Coping with Diverticulitis
Peter Cartwright

Coping with Dyspraxia
Jill Eckersley

Coping with Early-onset Dementia
Jill Eckersley

Coping with Endometriosis
Jill Eckersley and Dr Zara Aziz

Coping with Envy: Feeling at a disadvantage with friends and family
Dr Windy Dryden

Coping with Epilepsy
Dr Pamela Crawford and Fiona Marshall

Coping with Gout
Christine Craggs-Hinton

Coping with Guilt
Dr Windy Dryden

Coping with Headaches and Migraine
Alison Frith

Coping with Heartburn and Reflux
Dr Tom Smith

Coping with Life after Stroke
Dr Mareeni Raymond

Coping with Liver Disease
Mark Greener

Coping with Memory Problems
Dr Sallie Baxendale

Coping with Obsessive Compulsive Disorder
Professor Kevin Gournay, Rachel Piper and
Professor Paul Rogers

Coping with Pet Loss
Robin Grey

Coping with Phobias and Panic
Professor Kevin Gournay

Overcoming Common Problems Series

Overcoming Common Problems Series

Overcoming Common Problems

IBS

Dietary advice to calm your gut

ALEX GAZZOLA AND JULIE THOMPSON

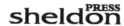
sheldon **PRESS**

First published in Great Britain in 2018

Sheldon Press
36 Causton Street
London SW1P 4ST
www.sheldonpress.co.uk

The authors and publisher have made every effort to ensure that the
external website and email addresses included in this book are correct and
up to date at the time of going to press. The authors and publisher are not
responsible for the content, quality or continuing accessibility of the sites.

British Library Cataloguing-in-Publication Data
A catalogue record for this book is available from the British Library

ISBN 978-1-84709-372-1
eBook ISBN 978-1-84709-373-8

Typeset by Fakenham Prepress Solutions, Fakenham, Norfolk NR21 8NN
First printed in Great Britain by Ashford Colour Press
Subsequently digitally printed in Great Britain

eBook by Fakenham Prepress Solutions, Fakenham, Norfolk NR21 8NN

Produced on paper from sustainable forests

Contents

Acknowledgements

The authors would like to thank: Vicky Grant, IBS researcher and patient advocate, who helped us to ensure this book is considerate to people with IBS; Jo Blackeley, clinical lead respiratory physiotherapist, who advised us with regard to physical activity and breathing; and Dr Sunil Sonwalkar, consultant gastroenterologist, for checking the accuracy of several medical points.

Note to the reader

This is not a medical book and is not intended to replace advice from your doctor. Consult your pharmacist or doctor if you believe you have any of the symptoms described and if you think you might need medical help.

Introduction: what is IBS?

Little about irritable bowel syndrome (IBS) is straightforward.

Let's start with the name itself. What does the word 'irritable' mean when applied to the bowel? Well, it tells us that the bowel has the potential to become irritated – or more sensitive – to certain foods and emotional stresses. Someone new to the name and unfamiliar with IBS may therefore assume the bowel is the sole organ affected by the condition, yet that is not necessarily true. Many with IBS experience headaches, depression, backache and other issues. Thus, the final word – 'syndrome', which means 'a collection of symptoms' – goes some way towards encapsulating the breadth of what IBS can be.

But is this name ideal or have its arguable weaknesses led to a widespread perception that it is a trivial condition, belittling those who live with it?

The term was first put forward in the 1940s, at a time when a variety of others were in use. 'Mucous colitis' – literally denoting inflammation of the colon with discharge of mucus – was around at least since the beginning of the last century and is certainly a harder-hitting name than 'irritable bowel syndrome' but it is inaccurate, as there is no obvious inflammation in IBS. 'Spastic colon' adequately described a colon (large bowel) vulnerable to spasms, but fell out of use in the UK and would now be considered unusable because of derogatory connotations. Others – such as 'windy colic', 'nervous stomach' and 'intestinal neurosis' – have cropped up from time to time and some such alternatives might still occasionally be used, especially in North America, or spotted in old medical journals.

What none of these alternative terms can adequately capture, however, is the multifaceted and variable nature of the condition. Nor can they do complete justice to the scope and scale of what people can go through.

So IBS is the term we have – the one that appears to have 'stuck' – but the continuing debates concerning the name indicate that, for some, it doesn't convey the seriousness of what they experience.

The variety of names used to describe IBS in decades past also shows the very real difficulty of succinctly characterizing and describing the condition – not least because there is much we don't know about it.

Unfortunately, to some extent, irritable bowel syndrome still has something of an identity crisis.

Defining IBS

Although the perception is beginning to be questioned by some experts, IBS is currently seen as a functional gastrointestinal disorder (FGID) – a disorder of how a part of the digestive system actually works – in which there is no obvious physical cause or abnormality.

In IBS, this disordered functioning involves gut contractions and movement – called 'motility' – and heightened gut sensations – called 'visceral hypersensitivity'.

It is characterized by such possible symptoms as lower abdominal pain or cramps, bloating or swelling in the belly, irregular or disordered bowel habits, excessive wind, sudden urgency to use the bathroom and, every now and again, incontinence. There may be diarrhoea or constipation or, indeed, both occurring alternately.

The severity varies widely: symptoms range from a minor inconvenience from time to time to being extremely socially restricting, having a profound impact on physical and mental well-being, week in, week out.

It can affect both sexes, though more women than men have IBS, and all ages, though it tends to manifest itself in early adulthood. We all occasionally experience at least some symptoms characteristic of IBS during our lives, but upwards of 12 per cent of Western populations either have medically diagnosed IBS or would fulfil the diagnostic criteria for the disease were they to be medically investigated. In the UK, that figure translates to at least six million people, many managing on their own.

What are the causes of IBS?

The answer to this is not straightforward either. We just don't yet know.

It may be the collection of symptoms that characterize IBS have more than one cause, and this is why people's experiences and responses to treatments vary so widely.

Some are diagnosed after a bout of gastroenteritis or food poisoning – this is called post-infectious IBS (IBS-PI). This may follow from an infection with the bacterium *Clostridium difficile* – common in those who have taken a course of certain antibiotics, such as penicillins – or from campylobacter bacteria, which are the most common cause of food poisoning, typically resulting from eating undercooked or raw chicken.

IBS is more prevalent in those who have joint hypermobility syndrome (JHS) – in which an individual's joints are looser, more supple or mobile than is the norm – because this condition can weaken digestive muscles; and also in Ehlers–Danlos Syndrome (EDS) – a genetic condition where collagen in the body's connective tissues is weaker than usual, which has an impact on the functioning of the digestive tract.

It has been associated with atopy – that is, a tendency towards allergic disease (such as asthma, eczema, hay fever) – and we know that a quarter of those with IBS have an atopic condition.

It can coexist with other chronic syndromes such as fibromyalgia (which causes widespread muscular pain) or systemic exertion intolerance disease (SEID; previously known as chronic fatigue syndrome or CFS) – in which people experience debilitating exhaustion – and it can also occur with other chronic gut disorders, such as inflammatory bowel disease or coeliac disease (autoimmune gluten hypersensitivity).

Additionally, we know that some people with mental health conditions and those recovering from an eating disorder or who have undergone traumatic life events, childhood bullying or stressful personal upheavals are more prone to IBS than the general population.

Often it is an illness without an obvious cause, but the factors known to be involved in triggering symptoms are diet and stress.

What you eat and how you feel or, to put it in a catchier way, food and mood.

The brain–gut axis

There is a strong neurological connection between the brain and the gut: a two-way biochemical channel of communication that appears to be at the core of IBS.

Essentially, this 'brain–gut axis' manages and regulates healthy digestive functioning for you so that in an ideal world, when this messaging system is working well, you are unaware of almost all aspects of it, such as the uptake of nutrients or the movement of food and waste matter through the intestine. In IBS, however, these signals may 'misfire': the interaction between brain and gut may be disrupted; the system malfunctions. The result may be abnormal gut motility and increased hypersensitivity.

Some 'brain-to-gut' scenarios will be familiar to all of us. Feelings of fear and stress can easily transfer to the bowel and manifest as a sudden increased urgency to use the toilet. The language we use on such occasions is testament to an awareness of our body's physical response to psychological factors: we may feel 'gutted' when the team we support suffers a difficult defeat; when we're frustrated or angry we may 'bellyache'; someone deeply upset may describe feeling 'sick to the pit of my stomach'.

Can symptoms arise the other way around – 'gut to brain'? Of course. When we eat a large meal, signals travel to relay a sense of satisfaction and relaxation, but perhaps lethargy and nausea result if we have slightly overdone it. We know that oversensitivity in the gut can be and is relayed to the brain and manifests as abdominal pain. Also, although we know that what we eat can have an impact on our mood, the question as to whether or not gut activity can affect our deeper psychological state is more complex.

And that could involve a third 'party' . . .

The microbiome

The bowel is not a sterile environment, and neither is it meant to be. Instead, it is home to vast colonies of bacteria, collectively known as the 'microbiome'.

Most of these gut bacteria are good for us; some, not so good. The good bacteria provide us with vital functions: they synthesize some vitamins, help with digestive processes and metabolic functions, help protect against allergy and inflammation and, importantly, keep the bad bacteria in check so they cannot establish themselves in quantities that impact negatively on health. They also help with digestive and metabolic functions – functions that are found to be abnormal in research animals bred 'sterile', with no microbiome.

The balance of bacteria can be affected by such factors as the foods we eat. We know that a high-fat or low-fibre diet can change the microbiome, for instance. We also know that a high-calorie diet is associated with a reduced diversity of gut bacteria, while a low-calorie diet improves the diversity – although we don't know why this might be. Certain foods – such as bananas, onions, wheat – contain prebiotics: sugars that good bacteria thrive on and therefore encourage their proliferation.

Also, the microbiome can be negatively affected by drugs and oral antibiotics, surgery, pregnancy, sleep dysfunction or disturbance, viral infections and other pathogens that get into the body.

There are potential consequences to any destabilization of the health of the microbiome. Studies on mice have shown that such changes can lower pain thresholds and speed up intestinal transit – both considered relevant in IBS.

The microbiome has an effect on intestinal permeability – that is, how easily or efficiently nutrients and salts from the gut's contents can be absorbed into the body through the gut wall and influence the immune system. This diffusion or absorption is important, so that nutrients can pass into the bloodstream, but excessive gut permeability may activate the immune system and lead to inflammation, both at a local level and potentially elsewhere in the body. The bacterial components themselves can trigger an immune response too.

Researchers also know that stress can alter the microbiome. Can this work in reverse? In other words, can an altered microbiome induce stress? One modest study found that a stool sample taken from a very anxious IBS patient, when transferred into rats, could induce anxiety in the animals, which may suggest that the microbiome could influence the brain and behaviour. We also know that this, in turn, can affect the gut . . . It can be a vicious circle.

So which might come first in such a scenario? A problem with the gut, with the microbiome or with the mind? That's a chicken-and-egg question to which there may be several answers.

The big picture

Not all the studies that have looked into these fascinating areas have been on humans and some of the ideas put forward in current discussions concerning IBS remain speculative. Research is continuing to unpick the complex nature of this syndrome. Ultimately, we may discover that IBS turns out to be a number of distinct conditions and it may need another 'rebrand' to account for what the research reveals.

For now, the microbiome–gut–brain axis is a good model for us to use, as these are the three key 'centres' of IBS.

It's also important to recognize that the bowel is full of nerves and could be argued to have its own 'brain' too. If the thought of IBS at least partly being in the brain worries you, though, we should stress that this is not the same as saying it is in the mind or in the imagination – which it certainly is not.

IBS is multifactorial, with the brain, central nervous system, gut, gut bacteria, our immune system and inflammatory responses all potentially involved. These are themes we will be dipping in and out of throughout this book.

How this book will help

So what of this book? How will it support you on your IBS journey?

Perhaps you have picked it up because you have recently been diagnosed with IBS and might be wondering whether or not changing your diet and lifestyle can help reduce symptoms. If so, you'll know that diagnosis is not a straightforward process and perhaps the advice dietitians give for IBS has changed recently and can be confusing – particularly when it is contradicted on some internet sites or by alternative therapists. We will help you to understand your IBS and how diet can be manipulated with the help of a dietitian to effectively manage your symptoms.

If you haven't been diagnosed, you might be wondering whether or not the symptoms you are having are down to IBS. It's important to *never* self-diagnose. See your doctor in the first instance, as it is necessary to rule out other medical conditions before IBS is considered as a diagnosis. We will guide you through that process and tell you what might be involved.

Although the focus here will be on food and diet, we will also consider healthy lifestyle issues and practical considerations, such as shopping and eating out. We hope that the Further reading and Useful addresses sections at the back of the book, as well as links elsewhere in the book, will be helpful in pointing you towards other reliable sources of information and useful products and services.

We don't intend to replace the treatment or personal advice of your GP, dietitian or gastroenterologist, but hope you will find the book to be a support and source of reference alongside the specialist care you receive from these qualified healthcare providers.

Throughout, we will focus on evidence – what we know about IBS – and make clear when aspects are less certain. Be suspicious of the advice given by unorthodox practitioners who may also try to sell you miracle solutions, allergy tests or special supplements for your IBS – occasionally we will warn you about them. Our advice is drawn from what unbiased, genuine experts with no secondary agenda believe to be true.

We wish you well on your journey.

1

Digestion: an introduction

Hidden within our bodies, the bowel is an enigmatic organ, and the business of digestion it undertakes, in partnership with the rest of the digestive system, can be equally mysterious to many of us.

Understanding both how digestion works when it works well, and how it goes wrong when it doesn't work so well, can be enormously beneficial and confidence-building. It can help you to look after your gut health during good times and take appropriate action at other times – as well as help reassure you that it is highly unlikely anything serious is the matter. Anybody's digestive system can malfunction from time to time. Worrying about IBS is not good for IBS. Knowledge can ease those worries.

So let's take a look at the 'inside' story . . .

What is digestion?

Most of the food we eat is of no use to the body in the form in which it is consumed.

In order for it to be of value, it must be broken down into smaller constituents that the body can then absorb and reassemble to suit its own needs – for instance, to build new cells or to nourish and fuel existing ones.

This breaking down of food is called 'digestion'.

The whole process occurs in the digestive tract (or alimentary canal): the tube that starts at your mouth, takes in the oesophagus (gullet), stomach and small and large intestines, and ends – up to ten metres later – at your bottom.

The agents that break down food into simpler molecules are called 'digestive enzymes'. Many of the enzymes and chemicals required for digestion are produced in the salivary glands, the liver, the gall bladder and the pancreas – vital organs that, together with the digestive tract, form the entire digestive system.

Which foods does the body need?

Foods provide the body with nutrients – the dietary components that we need to survive.

Proteins, carbohydrates, fats, vitamins, minerals, fibre and water are all required. Proteins, carbohydrates and fats are referred to as 'macronutrients', because they are needed in relatively high quantities; vitamins and minerals are referred to as 'micronutrients', as only modest or trace amounts are needed.

Proteins

These are provided mostly by meats, fish, eggs, grains, nuts and dairy products. The body breaks proteins down into peptides and amino acids before it can assimilate them and use them to build muscle, skin and other new cells.

Carbohydrates

'Complex carbohydrates' (starches) are found in breads, pasta, whole grains, pulses, fruits and vegetables.

'Simple carbohydrates' (sugars) are found in dairy products, fruit, vegetables and refined sweet products.

Unless already in their simplest state, all carbohydrates must be reduced to their constituent molecular units by enzymes before the body can efficiently use them as a source of energy.

Some carbohydrates – the fibre – can't be broken down as we don't produce the necessary enzymes. Bacteria in the gut can ferment some of these starches and sugars, and we will learn more about these 'fermentable carbohydrates' – called 'FODMAPs' – later.

Fats

These are found in meat, fish, eggs, nuts, butter and oils. The body breaks down fat into glycerol and fatty acids. These are important for healthy nerves, hormones, hair, skin and as a storable energy source.

Vitamins and minerals

These are present in virtually all foods and are required in modest amounts for a diversity of complex biological processes, from the formation of bone to the regulation of the cardiovascular system.

Fibre

Strictly speaking, this is a form of indigestible carbohydrate found in all plant foods. The terms 'soluble fibre' and 'insoluble fibre' are often used, which mean they either dissolve in water or they don't. In reality, plant foods contain *both* types of fibre and although experts have suggested that the terms should be phased out, they are still widely used, so an explanation of them is useful.

- **Insoluble fibre** is found in wholegrain products and the skins of fruits. It helps maintain digestive health.
- **Soluble fibre** is found in oats, beans, nuts and soft fruits. It also helps maintain a healthy bowel, but protects against heart disease and other long-term health issues too.

Again, our gut bacteria can help digest some of these fibres for us but not all.

Water

Arguably the most essential nutrient of all, as without it we would die within days. Every essential chemical process in the body occurs in its presence.

What happens in digestion?

From mouth to bottom, the digestive tract is essentially a long tube, acting as a selectively permeable barrier between the body and the tract's internal environment. Muscles in the tract stretch and contract to squeeze and propel food through – a process called 'peristalsis'. The tract's key role is to absorb the nutrients the body needs from the foods we eat. It is rich in nerves and has its own 'brain' – the 'enteric nervous system' – to help keep everything moving as it should.

Let's look at the process, stage by stage (see Figure 1.1).

The mouth

The very act of smelling food stimulates the salivary glands to produce saliva and the stomach to prepare to receive food before you even take your first bite. The mouth is the pleasure centre of taste and where digestion begins. Our teeth, honed by natural

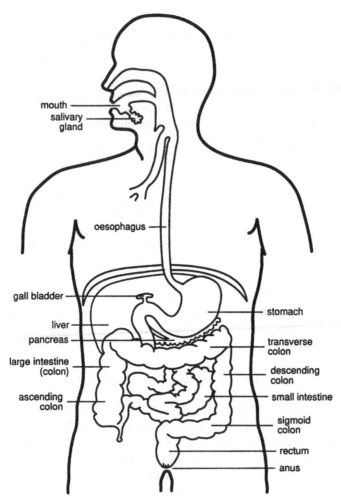

Figure 1.1 The digestive system

selection over millennia, are ideal for an omnivorous diet of both meat and plants. Chewing exposes more of our food's surface area to our digestive enzymes, which helps with digestion. Saliva lubricates food, making it easier to swallow, and contains an enzyme called 'amylase', which starts to break down carbohydrates into sugars.

The oesophagus (gullet)

At around 25 cm long, this flexible, muscular tube runs from our throat to our stomach. It takes several seconds for food to travel down the oesophagus into the stomach by peristalsis.

The stomach

This J-shaped organ receives food and liquid from the mouth via the gullet.

It secretes hydrochloric acid, to sterilize food and help break down protein, as well as other digestive enzymes, such as pepsin and lipase, which advance the digestion of protein and fats, respectively.

With its muscular wall, the stomach moves in waves to mix food and help break it down into smaller particles.

Food is usually in the stomach for an hour or more, but the length of time is determined by the make-up of the food – meals rich in fats, proteins and fibre remaining there for longer.

Small bowel

The small bowel or small intestine has three parts – the duodenum, the jejunum and the ileum. Although it is long, at about six metres, it is narrow. This is where digestion and food absorption take place in earnest.

The short duodenum receives food from the stomach and also bile from the liver and gall bladder, which helps to emulsify fats, and various enzymes from the pancreas, to help digest fats, protein and carbohydrates.

From the duodenum, food is pushed into the jejunum. Its mucous membranes secrete a mix of enzymes to further assist digestion. Here, some fats and amino acids, as well as simple sugars and vitamins, are absorbed.

Food is then pushed into the ileum, which absorbs water-soluble vitamins, amino acids, cholesterol and some salts.

The longer jejunum and ileum are coiled, and their inner walls are covered with tiny finger-like projections called 'villi' that increase the available surface area for the absorption of nutrients approximately to the size of a tennis court.

Usually food stays in the small intestine for a few hours only. At the end of the ileum is the ileocaecal valve, the main purpose of which is to prevent 'backflow' from the large bowel on the other side.

The large bowel

This is also called the 'large intestine' or 'colon' and there are four parts to it: the ascending colon, transverse colon, descending colon and sigmoid colon.

The ascending colon receives what is left over from the digestive processes that have taken place in the small intestine and begins the process of manufacturing stools from them. These are later passed out of the body in a process that can take a day or more.

As in the small bowel, the lining of the large bowel hosts bacteria, but on a much bigger scale. At any time, each of us has about a kilo or more of them in the colon. These help produce energy and some vital micronutrients and fatty acids by digesting starches and fibre.

As these contents are squeezed through, the bowel absorbs water, along with some simple nutrients, such as mineral salts. The developing stool gradually changes from liquid to relatively solid. Once it reaches the descending colon, it is almost fully formed.

The rectum

Stool from the descending colon collects in the rectum. When a sufficient quantity is present, an alert is sent to the brain that the rectum is ready to be emptied.

The anus

This is the opening to the end of the digestive tract where the formed stool leaves the body, rounding off the process of digestion.

Bowel reflexes

A 'reflex' is a movement over which we have no control and that occurs in response to a stimulus. There are many bowel reflexes and, given that disordered movements of the bowel are common in IBS, it is useful to understand what these might be.

The gastrocolic reflex

If the stomach is stretched after the consumption of a sizeable meal, this reflex can be triggered. Its effect is to speed up the movement of content through the bowel, leading to immediate diarrhoea for people with a sensitive bowel. This may leave you feeling that a certain food has resulted in the diarrhoea and you may be sensitive to it, but it may be down to the gastrocolic reflex. This may sometimes be due to the quantity of fats in what you've eaten, not a specific food intolerance.

Duodenal colic reflex

This is caused by distention in the duodenum, which can also result in speeding up movement of bowel contents, with similar results to the triggering of the gastrocolic reflex.

The ileocaecal reflex

This is triggered by distension of the ileum, increasing movement of contents through the ileocaecal valve. If the colon is full, the ileocaecal valve closes to prevent backflow of large bowel contents into the small bowel.

Digestive symptoms

We all experience digestive symptoms on a daily basis, or at least the common sensations that occur naturally as a consequence of digestive processes. Some we may barely register, while others may be more noticeable and a few problematic. Here we look at some of the most frequent.

Burping or belching

More formally known as 'ructus', this is the release of gas in the stomach through the mouth. It may be due to the air you swallow naturally as you eat – talking as you eat and eating fast or 'on the go' may mean you swallow more air. Fizzy drinks introduce gas too. You may also get hiccups if you swallow air or gas. In some, excessive burping may be a sign of a stomach ulcer or problem with your gall bladder.

Indigestion and heartburn

Medically termed 'dyspepsia', indigestion is discomfort in your tummy that usually comes after you've eaten food – often too fast or too much or food which is too hot or cold. Eating late at night, when standing up or when restless may bring on symptoms. It may also be related to stress, an irregular or erratic eating routine, certain medication, pregnancy, being overweight, smoking and tight clothing.

Heartburn or acid reflux is caused by acid in the stomach escaping up the gullet, sometimes reaching the back of the throat, causing a burning feeling. Indigestion and heartburn can also be instigated by a bacterial infection of the stomach, caused by a bacterium called *H. pylori*, which your doctor can check for if it is suspected.

Some foods may make both indigestion and heartburn worse. These include spicy foods, onions, tomatoes, fruit juices, chocolate, mint or mint tea, caffeinated drinks and alcohol.

Borborygmi

These are the rumbles or gurgles we all hear coming from our tummies from time to time. These are caused by the muscular contractions of the digestive tract when food or liquid is present. They are perfectly normal and usually much louder to you than anyone else! A 'growling' tummy may also signify hunger.

Flatulence and gas

It is normal to produce and pass gas. Those who say they don't are probably being economical with the truth! The average human passes gas up to 20 times a day.

Gas is a by-product of the fermentation of sugars by gut bacteria. Swallowed air can also contribute to increased levels, which can build up in the bowel if not released regularly. A normal quantity of gas in the large bowel is 100–200 ml. This may be a mix of methane, hydrogen, nitrogen and small amounts of oxygen and carbon dioxide.

Certain foods, including beans, lentils and pulses, sprouts and cauliflower, are notorious for causing gas. Its unpleasant odour can be the result of the sulphurous compounds present in certain amino acids commonly found in these and other foods, including meat, eggs, broccoli and onions. You shouldn't avoid these foods, as some are important for health, but if excess gas is a problem, cutting back can sometimes help. Lactose intolerance may increase gas too. We will be returning to all this later.

Bloating and distension

Bloating is a feeling of fullness and pressure in the abdomen. Some people with bloating will also experience distension – this is a marked increase in waist size.

Overeating, eating too fast and rich and fatty food can all increase the risk of bloating. Other culprits are fizzy drinks. Drinking through a straw and chewing gum can both increase the amount of air you swallow. Some of the foods that increase gas production may also be implicated.

Diarrhoea

This is passing looser than normal or very frequent stools.

Short-term diarrhoea is often caused by bacterial or viral infection or antibiotics and other medications.

Some foods are 'osmotically active', meaning they draw water from the body into the bowel as they pass through, which may increase the likelihood of diarrhoea. Fruit juice in large quantities is one such food, as the fructose (fruit sugar) in such amounts can have this effect.

Occasionally people may experience a temporary lactose intolerance after an episode of gastroenteritis and this can cause diarrhoea. This can improve, but if lactose intolerance persists for more than a few months, you should see your GP. More persistent episodes of diarrhoea may indicate IBS or, more rarely, some disorders or diseases of the bowel.

Constipation

This refers to the difficulty or infrequency of passing a stool or having to strain on the toilet. Hard, lumpy stools are common in those with constipation, as is a feeling of incomplete emptying of the bowel when managing to pass something.

It may be caused by a number of dietary factors, such as eating irregular meals, a low-fibre diet, an over-reliance on highly refined foods, low fluid intake or an abrupt change in diet.

A change of routine may trigger temporary constipation, as might stress and anxiety, lack of exercise, or regularly ignoring the urge to empty your bowel.

Constipation can also be a consequence of chronic slow transit of contents through the large bowel, a disorder of colonic and ano-rectal motility.

Stool colour

Can the colour of your poo indicate a medical problem? The answer is 'Yes, possibly', although food and medications can sometimes cause a colour change to your stools. A mid-brown stool is normal.

Green
This can be caused by changes in gut bacteria, diarrhoea or consumption of large amounts of green vegetables, including in green smoothies.

Red or purple
This can be caused by beetroot, cranberry or red food dye consumption or, if you have not consumed these foods, can be an indication of bleeding lower down in the digestive tract. If it is bright red, the change could be due to haemorrhoids, which should be referred to your doctor.

Grey
This might indicate a problem with your pancreas or a blockage of the tubes from the gall bladder and pancreas by a gallstone. See your doctor at once.

Black
This can be caused by iron tablets and bismuth-containing medications (such as Pepto-Bismol). It could indicate bleeding in the digestive tract. If the stool is smelly and has a tarry consistency, see a doctor urgently.

Yellow
This could be caused by excessive fat in the stool and can occur with IBS. It may also signify poor absorption of fat. If this is a new symptom and you are losing weight, then see your doctor. It can also result from consuming high-fat foods while taking the medication orlistat, which causes fat malabsorption.

2

Diagnosing IBS

Because there are no known physical abnormalities to detect in IBS, there are no tests available on the NHS that can confirm you have it. You will be assessed on the basis of the types of symptoms you have been experiencing.

Symptoms

There are many symptoms associated with IBS. All people will experience some but not all of them, and with varying severity.

IBS symptoms associated with the bowel

- Diarrhoea and/or constipation – sometimes alternating.
- Changes in your normal bowel habits.
- Pain, discomfort or cramps in your lower abdomen, sometimes preceding passing a stool.
- Urgency to use the bathroom – and perhaps incontinence.
- A feeling of incomplete emptying after passing a stool.
- Bloating and swelling of your belly.
- Excessive wind (flatulence).
- Passing mucus from your bottom.

IBS symptoms not associated with the bowel

- Backache – especially lower back pain.
- Muscular pains.
- Lethargy or lack of energy.
- Anxiety or depression.
- Lack of appetite.
- Pain during sex.
- Urgency to pass urine or waking up to pass urine at night.
- Nausea and digestive issues, such as heartburn.

Symptoms not usually associated with IBS

- Weight loss.
- Bleeding from your bottom.
- Abdominal pain waking you at night.
- High temperature.
- Fever.

Seeing your doctor

There can be a natural reticence, not wishing to 'bother' your doctor with something that you may fear he or she might consider trivial or with something you may have been living and 'getting by' with for some time. Furthermore, the embarrassment caused in discussing the bowel can make people feel uncomfortable.

Be reassured that no issue at all is too trivial for your doctor. It is worth making an appointment even for mild symptoms, for both the medical profession's sake and yours. It is more efficient and cost-effective to catch any issue as soon as possible, and you are likely to get a better outcome if you are treated early, should any treatment be needed.

It goes without saying that if you are worried, you *must* make an appointment with your GP, if only for reassurance.

It may help to make notes of what you wish to discuss ahead of the appointment and take them with you. Also, keep a record of your symptoms before you go or keep a symptom or food and symptom diary for a week (see Appendix 1). This is especially helpful, as we tend to properly recall only the most vivid or recent events, so keeping a diary helps us record things that may seem minor, but a doctor might recognize as significant.

Bristol Stool Form Scale

More commonly referred to as the Bristol Stool Chart, this is a chart of seven different 'categories' of typical stools, shown pictorially. Types one and two indicate constipation, types three and four indicate a normal stool form and types five to seven indicate diarrhoea. The chart can help if you don't like to talk about the bowel and poo – you can just point! You can find it at <www.hct.nhs.uk/media/1067/bristol-stool-chart.pdf>.

The consultation

The ultimate aim of any consultation is to establish the presence or absence of a condition or illness and determine a therapy or treatment for any which is found. Your doctor will probably focus on your symptom history and current symptom profile. He or she will do this by listening to what you have to say about your health and asking questions, in particular about the pain and discomfort you may be experiencing and the impact symptoms are having on your day-to-day life – such as if they prevent you from leaving your home.

All health practitioners get used to talking about symptoms and some may forget to ask if you feel comfortable doing so. Let your practitioner know if you find it difficult. Having kept a detailed diary in advance of your appointment can help with issues you may feel shy about voicing, such as incontinence. If you book your appointment online, you could give your main symptoms in the 'reason for visit' section.

Your doctor may ask about your diet and lifestyle, and may ask you to lie down to feel your tummy. You may also be asked about your stress and anxiety levels or to complete a questionnaire designed to get an idea of how stress may affect your day-to-day life.

Might it be IBS?

Healthcare professionals are advised to consider assessing for IBS if someone presents with one or more of the following 'ABC' symptoms over the last six months:

- abdominal pain
- bloating
- change in bowel habits.

Furthermore, they will consider a diagnosis of IBS if any pain or discomfort is either relieved by pooing or associated with altered bowel frequency or stool form, and is accompanied by two or more of these symptoms:

- altered passing of stool (straining, urgency, incomplete emptying of the bowel);

- bloating, distension, tension;
- symptoms made worse by eating;
- passing mucus from the bottom.

Might it be something else?

Because the symptoms typically associated with IBS can also be associated with other conditions or diseases, blood tests can rule these out. All the following should be performed.

Full blood count (FBC)

This is a common test that medics use as a general health screen and to look for common conditions such as anaemia.

Erythrocyte sedimentation rate (ESR) and C-reactive protein (CRP)

ESR examines the behaviour of your red blood cells, in order to determine whether or not you may have an inflammatory disorder or inflammation in the body. Raised levels of CRP also indicate inflammation. Inflammatory bowel disorders such as Crohn's disease or ulcerative colitis can sometimes be mistaken for IBS.

Coeliac disease tests

Raised levels of certain antibodies (called EMA and tTG) strongly indicate possible coeliac disease – which is an autoimmune condition triggered by gluten in the diet. Gluten is found in wheat, rye, barley and some oats, and most products made from them. This test assumes you have been following a gluten-containing diet. If you have excluded gluten – which you should never do without medical advice – your doctor may ask you to reintroduce it for six weeks ahead of the test.

A test for genes called HLA-DQ2 or HLA-DQ8 – which are present in all people with coeliac disease but also many people without – may be performed in certain circumstances, such as if the antibody tests are borderline or uncertain.

Ovarian cancer and endometriosis

These can cause vague symptoms that are similar to those of IBS. Ovarian cancer is very rare in women under 60 and can be tested for via a CA125 blood test, in addition to other investigations, such as an ultrasound or computerized tomography (CT) scan. Some women with underlying endometriosis have raised CA125 levels, so this is not something to be overly alarmed about.

Endometriosis, which typically affects women during menstruation, is where cells lining the womb migrate and deposit at other sites in the body, causing inflammation and pain. This is a bit of a challenge to diagnose and can only be definitively identified by carrying out a laparoscopy (a tiny camera is inserted into the abdomen under general anaesthetic).

Although it is common to experience pain and a worsening of IBS symptoms around the time of your period (see page 106), if you have severe abdominal pain, your doctor may refer you to a gynaecologist. Other symptoms of endometriosis are pain on opening your bowel and deep pelvic pain during sex.

Endometriosis UK offers a useful pain diary, available via the organization's website (<www.endometriosis-uk.org>), which you might want to consider using before you visit your GP.

Women can be diagnosed as having both endometriosis and IBS.

Secondary care (hospital) investigations

If, for instance, any of the blood tests described above indicate the possibility of IBS or another condition, your doctor may refer you for further tests, perhaps with a gastroenterologist (a doctor specializing in the gut). He or she may also refer you to a specialist if there are any so-called 'red flag' indicators. These are:

- unexplained and unintentional weight loss;
- bleeding from the bottom or blood in stools;
- a family history of cancer of the bowel;
- abdominal or rectal masses – growths in the lower abdomen or bowel, should your doctor suspect you have them after a physical examination;
- in women, a family history of cancer of the ovaries (for which

your doctor may first order a test for levels of CA125 – a protein in the blood that can be associated with ovarian cancer; see box on page 15);

• in the over 60s, a change in bowel habits to loose or more frequent stools, lasting more than six weeks.

Some possible investigations include those described below. Remember that these will only occasionally be needed and not everyone being investigated for IBS will require one or more of them.

Ultrasound

This test uses sound waves to look at the abdomen, gall bladder and liver, and ovaries in women.

Abdominal X-ray

This is an X-ray of the abdomen of internal organs and structures, usually requested for symptoms of abdominal pain, bloating, nausea and vomiting.

Gastroscopy

This uses a narrow tube with a camera at the tip to view the upper digestive system – the oesophagus, stomach and duodenum. It can be used to look for cancers, Barrett's oesophagus (abnormal cells lining the oesophagus, caused by acid reflux), oesophagitis (inflamed gullet), gastritis (inflamed stomach), duodenitis (inflamed small bowel), hiatus hernia, and stomach and duodenal ulcers.

If you have raised coeliac disease antibodies (see page 14), you may be advised to undergo an endoscopy and biopsy of the small bowel. In this procedure, a tube with a device on the end is passed through the mouth into your small bowel via your stomach in order to obtain small samples of bowel lining. These are then examined in a laboratory for evidence of the characteristic erosion caused by gluten.

Colonoscopy

A colonoscopy is similar to a gastroscopy, but instead the device is passed into the body via the anus to examine the lining of the large intestine. It will look for polyps (non-cancerous growths from the bowel wall), diverticulosis (pouches protruding through the wall of the large bowel), inflammatory bowel disease and cancer. You might be referred for this test if you have anaemia, are over 55, have a change in usual bowel habits or weight loss or are bleeding via the rectum.

Small bowel meal

This is a series of examinations of the small intestine. You will be asked to swallow a white contrast drink that shows up under X-ray and can indicate Crohn's disease and any tumours.

Faecal calprotectin

This recently developed stool test identifies inflammation in the bowel. It may be used by your GP, but is more likely to be used in the hospital setting. It is more accurate than the ESR as it is targeted to look for inflammation present in inflammatory bowel disease.

Other investigations

Other investigations may include those described below.

Bile acid malabsorption test

Bile acid, which is made by the liver and stored in the gall bladder, emulsifies fats and helps them to be absorbed. The gall bladder contracts and releases bile acid into the small intestine in response to meals. It can contract at other times too. Any bile left after fats have been digested is absorbed at the end of the small intestine.

If you have had your gall bladder removed, the bile dribbles into the digestive tract all the time. Any bile acid not absorbed in the small bowel reaches the large bowel, the lining of which can be irritated as a consequence. This is very uncomfortable and results in watery diarrhoea.

Ten per cent of people without a gall bladder will suffer from diarrhoea, and around a quarter of people with diarrhoea-dominant IBS have bile acid malabsorption. If you are getting up frequently at night to empty your bowel and your stools are frequent and watery, talk to your doctor about a possible referral for bile acid malabsorption testing – called SeHCAT. More commonly, though, if bile acid malabsorption is suspected, your GP may suggest you try Questran, colestipol or colesevelam – medications to treat the diarrhoea.

Hydrogen breath testing

This is usually used to test for lactose intolerance.

Lactose is the sugar that naturally occurs in milk and can be found in many dairy products. Our bodies produce an enzyme called lactase that digests lactose, but levels may be low or compromised in some people, which means lactose digestion cannot take place.

When this happens, gut bacteria ferment the sugar and diarrhoea can result. As a consequence of this fermentation, hydrogen is produced and this passes through the bowel wall into the blood, later showing up in your breath. The test detects this.

If you feel you have a problem with lactose, then you could make a change to lactose-free milks, yogurt and cheeses for two to four weeks (these products have the same level of calcium as cow's milk) and see if the symptoms resolve.

If the symptoms continue, then lactose intolerance is unlikely and you should reintroduce ordinary milk into your diet.

If they stop, as a simple test you could drink a glass of ordinary milk to see whether or not they return. If they do, then lactose intolerance is likely.

Your doctor may then refer you for hydrogen breath testing to confirm the suspicion. It involves measuring hydrogen in your breath, both before and after you consume a lactose solution.

Other than lactose intolerance, a hydrogen breath test may also be used to test for a more uncertain condition called small bowel or intestinal bacterial overgrowth (SBBO or SIBO).

Although the small bowel is usually almost free of bacteria, slow movement of food through the duodenum may result in bacteria colonizing it to a greater degree than is normal. This 'bacterial overgrowth' can lead to diarrhoea, flatulence, weight loss and weakness, which may underlie IBS, and so some doctors will consider it worthwhile investigating. Others, however, doubt the existence of SBBO and believe that a positive breath test for it merely reflects disordered intestinal transit speed (be it faster or slower than normal), which is common in IBS.

Breath tests may also be investigations a dietitian can order (including for other sugars), and we will return to them in Chapter 4.

H. pylori *bacteria test*

H. pylori is a bacterium that lives in the stomach and causes stomach ulcers and symptoms of indigestion, heartburn and reflux. This test may be requested if you still have symptoms of reflux despite trying medications and lifestyle modifications, have difficulty swallowing, are aged over 55 or have been experiencing reflux symptoms and weight loss.

There are two main tests for this:

- **urea breath test** you drink a solution that is broken down by *H. pylori* and your breath is then analysed;
- **stool antigen test** a sample of your poo is examined in a laboratory.

Giardiasis/bacterial stool test

Giardia are parasites that can cause diarrhoea and abdominal pain. Stool samples can be analysed in a laboratory for giardia cysts. Your doctor may also send a sample of your poo to test for bacteria that cause gastroenteritis.

Faecal elastase test

This test is likely to be considered if you are experiencing weight loss and severe pain and diarrhoea at night. It tests for an enzyme that is increased when the pancreas is not working properly and not producing digestive enzymes. A sample of poo will be analysed at a laboratory.

Non-coeliac gluten sensitivity investigations

A final possibility is this emerging condition, which has made the medical news in recent years. It is often abbreviated to NCGS, though some argue that it should be called non-coeliac wheat sensitivity (NCWS).

Some experts believe that, even in those without coeliac disease, gluten can cause similar symptoms and other issues, such as neurological symptoms, while others feel the evidence is lacking and suspect the culprits are, in fact, other components of wheat, such as FODMAPs or non-gluten proteins. It may turn out to be that some with NCGS/NCWS have a form of 'pre-coeliac' disease.

Some cases may be down to the 'nocebo effect' – roughly meaning that negative effects are caused by expecting the worst. In this case, the effect might manifest as feeling ill after consuming gluten due to the expectation that this will happen. The popularization of the gluten-free diet among celebrities as a means to weight loss or for the relief of bloating has given further support to the idea of NCGS among the wider public, but it is not yet fully proven scientifically. Research is continuing into this new disease entity, as more is needed to first prove its existence and then understand its mechanism.

Should you be referred to a gastroenterologist, NCGS may be considered – although a low-FODMAP diet is far more likely to benefit you (see Chapter 4).

Symptoms of NCGS can be similar to IBS, so it is challenging to distinguish the two as no test is yet available. They include abdominal pain, diarrhoea, headache, fatigue, depression and brain fog, joint pain and numbness.

A diagnosis would depend on first excluding the possibility of either coeliac disease or wheat allergy, followed by a positive gluten challenge – that is, relief of symptoms on a gluten-free diet, followed by the return of symptoms when gluten is reintroduced. This is challenging to undertake objectively and a dietitian should be involved.

Unvalidated tests

The methods of diagnosis discussed in this chapter are the only ones we know to be reliable and relevant. They are based on sound medical research and are available from your doctor. There exist other tests – available via private laboratories and alternative therapists, for example – that are unsubstantiated and considered unscientific by experts. Often, they come at a high price. We urge you to avoid all, as they can introduce confusion and doubt into your mind about your health and there is no good evidence that they work or are relevant.

While there are blood tests for food *allergies* that are useful, be aware that there are none for food *intolerances*. Some laboratories offer blood tests for food antibodies called IgG, under the premise that raised IgG levels indicate intolerance. That is not the case. Researchers and allergists believe IgG antibodies indicate *exposure* to foods, *not* intolerance.

Some alternative practitioners offer other means of food intolerance testing. These include applied kinesiology (which tests for reduced muscular strength when the person is given a food to hold), bio-resonance hair testing (a sample of the person's hair is analysed for supposed energy pattern imbalances and nutritional issues), cytotoxic testing (which exposes white blood cells to food extracts), pulse testing (which monitors pulse rate on oral exposure to a food) and electrodermal skin testing (which tests skin conductivity when a food is placed within an electrical circuit). None of these has any basis in science.

Often, and sometimes after performing such tests, alternative practitioners encourage the removal of wheat and milk to their clients and report a high success rate as a result. This is likely to be because both are high-FODMAP foods, which may provoke symptoms in many with IBS or food intolerances. It does not mean that the practitioners' diagnostic methods are reliable.

Unvalidated diagnoses

Practitioners may use unvalidated tests and other methods to diagnose you with conditions that modern medicine does not recognize.

One is ileocaecal valve syndrome, which is based on the proposition that a malfunctioning ileocaecal valve may cause allergies and IBS symptoms, yet there is no evidence for this or for the condition's existence.

Another is leaky gut syndrome, proposed by alternative health practitioners as a cause of conditions such as chronic fatigue, fibromyalgia, IBS and others. This is based on the idea that 'toxins' are absorbed into the blood via an excessively porous or 'leaky' gut, causing a variety of effects on health.

The cells lining the large bowel have junctions between them that in normal circumstances are 'tight'; the cells also produce a protective layer of mucus. This barrier allows the passage of small molecules (such as digested nutrients and salts), but prevents larger molecules, such as proteins, from passing through. Microbes have a role in keeping this barrier functioning well.

Hypersensitivity in the digestive tract is a cardinal symptom of IBS and the tight junctions can become more 'open', allowing proteins and microbes through. This is suspected of increasing sensitivity to normal reflexes and movement of contents through the digestive tract. This can occur with low levels of inflammation seen after gastroenteritis (food poisoning).

While we know that low levels of gut inflammation in IBS are possible, and this may make the gut 'leakier' to some extent, we *do not* have a specific treatment that we know is effective for increased gut permeability. This is still a somewhat controversial theory among some in the medical establishment, but is growing as a concept and research is continuing.

The supplements or herbal remedies the alternative practitioner may recommend may not be that effective as treatments. Instead, diet can help symptoms, as might probiotics to a small extent, but your dietitian or gastroenterologist are the best individuals to advise on this.

Confirming the IBS diagnosis

Much of this chapter is drawn from a guidance document published by the National Institute for Health and Care Excellence (NICE) on the diagnosis and management of IBS in adults. This is a recommended method that doctors should follow.

Diagnostic criteria

When certain causes of symptoms have been ruled out, a medic may use a diagnostic algorithm – such as the Rome Criteria, which you may hear your doctor mention or may come across in other contexts – to help him or her reach a conclusion in order to diagnose IBS. Some may instead use experience and instinct – with the support of exclusion tests – to confirm a suspicion of IBS.

Which IBS?

Although not all experts consider them particularly useful, there are several IBS subtypes that may describe the IBS you're diagnosed as having. Many individuals with IBS will alternate between these types over time. Even if you are not given a subtype, you will be aware of which you have and can still be confident in the accuracy of an IBS diagnosis.

- **IBS-C** constipation-predominant IBS (IBS type C), where constipation is the main symptom.
- **IBS-D** diarrhoea-predominant IBS (IBS type D), where diarrhoea is the main symptom.
- **IBS-A** 'alternating' IBS, where the person experiences both diarrhoea and constipation.
- **IBS-PI** post-infectious IBS, which may be diagnosed following an apparent bout of gastrointestinal infection – usually bacterial – followed by a sudden onset of IBS symptoms.
- **IBS-U** unclassified IBS, where the distinction is not clearly defined.

Accepting a diagnosis of IBS

For some people a diagnosis of IBS can often be preceded by an intensely frustrating process. You may have undergone myriad tests before your doctor reaches a conclusion that the problem is a functional one. If your symptoms have been severe, you may have been expecting and preparing for a disease diagnosis, not one of IBS.

This can result in various or mixed feelings, which is understandable. You may be relieved, but you may also feel the diagnosis doesn't adequately reflect the severity of your symptoms. You may be left in need of reassurance about your diagnosis and lacking confidence in being able to manage your symptoms going forward. You may also feel despondent that your doctor might consider the diagnosis 'good' because you don't have cancer or an inflammatory bowel disease.

Given that IBS is often described as a 'diagnosis of exclusion', this can further magnify any suspicion that your doctor isn't sure what is the matter with you, merely relieved that you don't have something considered more serious.

If you feel dissatisfied, you may understandably feel the urge to request further tests for what you fear may be an undetected problem, the discovery of which will justify your symptoms to yourself, your family and your doctor. Yet there are cases on record of individuals undergoing gall bladder removal surgery as a consequence of acute symptoms that are later discovered to be down to IBS. Thus, further invasive tests or treatments can result in side effects that might be unhelpful to your IBS in the long term.

A positive diagnosis

You may not view a diagnosis of IBS as 'positive', but it does mean you can be reassured that your doctor is satisfied and confident there is no other disease producing the symptoms you have been experiencing. Also, IBS, while certainly having a great impact on some people's quality of life, is not going to shorten your life or mean that you are at increased risk of future bowel disease or cancer.

Although the causes of IBS are not well understood, we do know what happens in the bowel to trigger symptoms and doctors are learning more and more about it. At the same time, new treatments continue to be developed. Your doctor can direct you towards many of these, which are available for you to try and may help manage your IBS in the long term.

IBS is very individual and the best person to know what is going to work for you is you, once you're aware of what is available to help. Learning about your IBS is an important part of the process of healing and will enable you to feel confident that you can manage it in the long term, help you come to terms with and accept your new situation and, ultimately, live your life to the full.

The patient–practitioner relationship

Something else that may affect how 'positively' you view the diagnosis is how it was given to you, which is important in establishing a basis from which to try treatments and empower yourself to manage symptoms. Ideally, your doctor should be fully confident in your diagnosis: 'We know for sure it is IBS, so let's look at what we can do to help.'

Occasionally, practitioners can appear to be a little dismissive of IBS. Remember, doctors are only human and they may not always deliver the news in the manner you would prefer. They may say, 'Oh, it's just IBS' or 'You'll be fine' or 'It's all in your mind – if you relax more, it'll get better.' They may wrongly assume that you are 'pleased' with your diagnosis – perhaps because it isn't cancer – when you know only too well there is nothing pleasing about being given a diagnosis of a life-long condition which may need careful management. You may feel helpless when faced with this attitude and disinclined to try treatments as a result.

Because it is so important for you to have a strong patient–practitioner relationship, based on trust, dignity and mutual respect, it is vital that you raise concerns with your practitioner. Most practitioners want to get the relationship right too.

In such a situation, however, you may feel unable to discuss concerns about your diagnosis with your doctor. If so, you can ask to see another doctor when you book your next appointment or you might find that you can work better with a different healthcare provider, such as a practice nurse, who may have more time to spend with you.

Most healthcare providers are naturally empathetic – this emotion is often what has driven them towards their profession – but some are more naturally so than others. If your practitioner is one of those who is less so, it does not necessarily mean that the standard of treatment is worse per se; in fact, some will work well with their practitioner in this situation.

It is, however, important that *you* feel confident in your care provision. The relationships between you, your doctor and other healthcare practitioners are important in achieving this confidence and moving forward with recommended treatment options with positivity.

IBS treatments

These can take a number of forms.

Lifestyle advice

There is some general lifestyle advice your doctor may give you or discuss with you. This may include:

- changes to your diet, such as adjusting fibre intake, which we will cover in Chapter 3, along with other simple healthy eating tips, and in many other cases, your doctor will refer you to a dietitian (see Chapter 4) for more advanced dietary recommendations, such as the low-FODMAP diet;

- looking after your emotional well-being and personal relationships (see Chapter 7);
- making time for relaxation and leisure activities, while also increasing your physical activity levels if they are low (see Chapter 8).

Therapies

These might include:

- talking therapies, counselling and cognitive behavioural therapy (see Chapter 7);
- biofeedback training, which may be useful for constipation, if it is due to outlet delay and for where the pelvic floor muscle coordination is not so good and the bowel cannot be opened without pressure or straining as it aims to teach people to recognize internal signs of relaxation and uses exercises to retrain the pelvic floor and relax the anal sphincter.

Drugs

Doctors may prescribe certain drugs, some of which are listed below.

- **For pain** Buscopan is a first-line medication, but also antispasmodic agents (Mebeverine, peppermint oil in capsules), linaclotide (for IBS-C), some probiotic supplements and tricyclic antidepressants (TCAs, if antispasmodic agents have failed).
- **For bloating** linaclotide (for IBS-C), some probiotic supplements, avoidance of bulking agents and certain fibre sources.
- **For constipation** laxatives (but not lactulose), bulking agents, stool softeners, stimulants, osmotics, linaclotide, tricyclic antidepressants (TCAs).
- **For diarrhoea** antimotility agents (loperamide being the first choice), antispasmodic agents.
- **For other symptoms** antibiotics, such as for SIBO or *H. pylori* infection.

3

Healthy eating

Symptoms of IBS are without doubt affected by what we eat and drink, and most people would like dietary solutions to these symptoms in preference to medication or other interventions.

Sometimes, changing your diet according to healthy eating guidelines can help with mild forms of IBS, and certainly not everyone needs to make drastic changes. This chapter looks at some simple healthy eating suggestions and adjustments.

Healthy eating

First, it's important to consider what we mean by healthy eating in practice. We hear so much in the media about good nutrition, sometimes contradictory or faddy, that it's hardly surprising many of us may be confused as to what we should be consuming.

The first principle of good nutrition is variety. Research shows many of us rely on just a few foods that we eat regularly, but we should eat a broad selection of grains, protein sources, vegetables and fruits to ensure we provide our bodies a wide variety of nutrients.

Freshly prepared meals, from whole ingredients, can be better for your IBS – but if you struggle to find time to prepare your own lunches and dinners, the stress of trying to do so may negatively affect your IBS, so compromises may have to be considered. Enlist the help of family members, if you can.

But so-called healthy eating may not *always* be helpful in IBS, and other advice in this chapter may be more helpful to you.

Dietary balance

What proportions of different foods should we eat to ensure our bodies receive the nutrients they need to keep us healthy?

Bread, rice, potatoes, pasta

At least a third of our daily diet should be complex wholegrain starchy carbohydrates – at least three portions per day.

Increasing fibre sources from wheat bran does not help IBS symptoms, so do not boost your intake of wholegrain wheat bread and wholegrain wheat breakfast cereals, for example. Choose alternatives to wheat such as rice bran, brown rice, oats and jacket potatoes.

Fruit and vegetables

This should comprise a third of our daily dietary intake. 'Five a day' advice is well known, but in the longer term up to ten may be better. Aim for five at first and go for a 'rainbow' of coloured fruit and vegetables, including ones that are purple, green, yellow, orange and red.

Milk and dairy foods

These foods should make up about a fifth of your intake – that is, in three portions a day (190 ml milk, 125 g yogurt or 30 g cheese is a portion).

These foods are important for your 700 mg a day calcium requirements.

If you follow a milk-free diet, ensure that your milk alternatives (such as soya milks) are fortified with calcium and vitamin D to ensure you do not miss out on these important nutrients.

Meat, fish, eggs, beans

This is also a fifth of your intake. Try to choose lower-fat versions of protein foods, unless you are underweight or losing weight, in which case seek medical advice.

Foods high in fat and/or sugar

Cakes, biscuits, confectionery, crisps and sugary drinks should only ever form a very small proportion of the diet, with no more than 5 per cent of our daily calories (around 100–125) from added sugars. Fructose-based sugars such as high-fructose corn syrup and fructose–glucose syrups can trigger symptoms in some people with IBS.

Weight and body mass index (BMI)

Although there is no evidence that being over- or underweight can result in IBS, if you wish to address any issues you may have with your weight you might consider either decreasing or increasing your calorie intake.

If you are overweight, a reduction of around 500 calories a day should result in a loss of up to 1 kilo a week. Apps such as My Fitness Pal can be useful, and NHS Choices offers a free 12-week weight loss programme (see the Useful addresses section for details).

Many people are underweight as a result of reluctance to eat due to symptoms of IBS. Increasing intake by at least 500 calories a day should lead to weight gain.

Your body mass index (BMI) can help determine whether you are underweight or overweight. Calculate it by dividing your weight in kilograms by your height in metres squared (your height in metres multiplied by itself) or see the NHS Healthy Weight calculator at <www.nhs.uk/Tools/Pages/Healthyweightcalculator.aspx>. The following list provides a useful guide.

- **Underweight** less than 20 kg/m^2
- **Healthy** 20–25 kg/m^2
- **Overweight** 25–30 kg/m^2
- **Obese** greater than 30 kg/m^2

In whichever situation you find yourself, a dietitian can offer guidance.

Tackling symptoms

Combined with the lifestyle advice and possible medication you've been advised to take via your doctor, some simple dietary advice may also further help ease symptoms.

If you have diarrhoea . . .

Diarrhoea is caused by fast transit of contents through the large bowel, due to rapid contractions. This can sometimes be caused by diet and medications (antibiotics, antihypertensives, antidepressants and others). Speak with your pharmacist or doctor if you think medications are a cause.

- Drink plenty of fluids.
- Have no more than one small glass of fruit juice daily (100 ml) and spread up to three portions of fruit throughout the day.
- Reduce daily intake of caffeine to no more than three cups of coffee.
- Reduce intake of sugar-free sweets and gum.
- Swap wholegrain breakfast cereals, bread and starchy foods to white or low-fibre varieties.
- Try lactose-free cow's milk instead of standard cow's milk.
- Reduce intake of cakes, biscuits and high-fat foods.

If you have constipation . . .

Constipation can be caused by a low intake of fluid and fibre and can, in some people, occur as a result of chronic poorly contracting gut or colonic inertia. It could also occur as a result of an outlet delay (when the pelvic floor muscles and anal sphincters fail to relax during defaecation) or hard stools with a normal functioning bowel. Other possibilities are certain medications (painkillers, blood pressure tablets and antidepressants – speak to your doctor or pharmacist if you suspect any of these), inactivity or medical conditions such as underactive thyroid.

- Drink plenty of fluids.
- Increase fibre intake with fruit, vegetables and wholegrain starchy foods such as oats, brown rice, potatoes with skins.
- Add a tablespoon of linseeds to soup, salad, yogurt or cereals.
- Increase fibre intake slowly to allow time for your bowel to adjust.
- Don't increase fibre intake with wheat bran as this could make symptoms worse.

If you suffer from bloating/flatulence . . .

Bloating – a feeling of fullness and pressure in the abdomen – is a common symptom and widely considered one of the most bothersome. It tends to get worse during the course of the day, and more women suffer than men.

It can sometimes, but not always, be caused by too much gas or by visceral hypersensitivity. People with IBS may have abnormal abdominal wall reflexes – possibly as a consequence of pain and subsequent awkward positioning of the body, which may explain the absence of symptoms on rising in the morning.

Bloating can also be as a result of abnormal handling of fluids within the small intestine, and fermentation. We will return to this subject in Chapter 4.

- Have no more than one small glass of fruit juice a day (100 ml), and no more than three portions of fruit, spread throughout the day.
- Reduce your intake of beans, broccoli, cabbage, cauliflower and sugar-free foods containing polyol sweeteners (such as sorbitol, maltitol, xylitol).
- Try lactose-free milk – it contains similar levels of calcium to standard milk.
- People with wind or bloating may find it helpful to eat oats (such as porridge or oat-based cereal) and linseeds.

Caffeine and coffee

Coffee stimulates bowel contractions, so if you consume strong coffee cutting back might help.

Further, the caffeine in coffee can disrupt sleep and increase anxiety, so reduction may be worth a try, especially if you also consume tea, chocolate and cola, which also contain caffeine.

Reduce intake slowly, as withdrawal symptoms (headache, irritability, drowsiness) may result if you abruptly stop caffeine intake.

Coffee contains many complex chemicals and we don't know if it is just the caffeine that triggers symptoms. Some people report reactions to decaffeinated coffee too.

Food	Approximate caffeine content
Coffee expresso (small cup)	200 mg
Coffee filter (1 cup)	140 mg
Coffee instant (1 cup)	100 mg
Energy drinks (250 ml)	80 mg
Tea (1 cup)	75 mg
Cola (330 ml)	25 mg
Chocolate (dark, 25 g)	20 mg
Chocolate (milk, 25 g)*	10 mg

*Also contains high levels of fat and lactose.

Levels of caffeine vary depending on the product. Note that pregnant women should consume no more than 200 mg per day. For IBS, the recommendations are to have no more than three cups of coffee per day.

Medication can contain caffeine to improve the effectiveness of the drug, and it can also be found in supplements. Do not stop taking medication, but discuss this with your doctor or pharmacist as there may be an alternative.

Fats

High intakes of fat can cause almost immediate diarrhoea through the gastrocolic reflex for some with digestive disorders. Sometimes reduction in the levels of fat consumed can be all that's required to reduce symptoms in mild IBS.

Labels should state the amount of total fat per 100 g. Consider both this figure and the portion size of the food. If you eat a large portion of a food containing a medium level of fat this might be enough to cause symptoms. Some manufacturers use a 'traffic light' system as a guide (see Table 3.1).

Fat is a high-calorie food component. Most people eat too much, but some fats are key to a healthy diet, providing essential fatty acids such as omega-3 oil and fat-soluble vitamins.

Reduce the amounts of cakes, biscuits, pastries and chocolate in your diet. Full fat cheese can be replaced with lower-fat versions, especially if you are overweight. Choose healthier fat options such as sunflower or olive oil, and olive oil-based spreads.

Eat one portion of oily fish per week, in the form of 100 g of salmon, pilchards, mackerel or sardines; if you are vegan, try walnuts and rapeseed, soya or linseed oils.

Table 3.1 The 'traffic light' labelling system

Level of fat	Quantity of fat	Colour of label
Low	Less than 3 g per 100 g	Green
Medium	Between 3 and 17.5 g per 100 g	Amber
High	Greater than 17.5 g per 100 g	Red

Chilli and spicy foods

These are commonly blamed for symptoms, usually because of their heat, but this may not be the cause for everyone. Spicy dishes often contain significant amounts of onion and garlic, which, as we shall see later, may be responsible. Try using chilli without onion and garlic in a dish to see if that helps.

Resistant starches

As their name suggests, these complex carbohydrates are resistant to digestion. They are commonly found in chilled foods, potato salad and reheated potato products such as oven chips, in toast and in reheated pasta and rice products. They may be added to processed foods to thicken or improve 'mouthfeel'.

IBS guidelines have for some time advised a reduction in the intake of resistant starch, but support for this has waned, and with other approaches most people will not have to directly modify their intake.

Food exclusion

Although in this chapter we tentatively suggest experimenting with some food swaps and with the restriction or increase of certain foods, it's unwise to make more drastic changes to your diet at this stage.

Some people's diets become excessively restricted with IBS, especially when they find symptoms are eased by not eating. Eating little is simply not sustainable.

Excluding food groups – such as all grains, all dairy products or all fruits – should never be undertaken independently of medical care. This can lead to malnutrition, which is only likely to lead to further digestive distress, creating a cycle of further restrictions and symptoms. Complete exclusion can also induce more sensitivity for some foods, occasionally making it more difficult to reintroduce important nutrients.

Remember: the type of food you eat may not be a problem, and you may not have a food intolerance. Investigating this is complicated, and should be done under the care of a dietitian. We will look at this in the next chapter.

Fibre

This is carbohydrate that is neither digested by nor absorbed into the body.

Previously, fibre intake modification was a mainstay treatment for IBS: less fibre for diarrhoea and more – including wheat bran – for those with constipation. We now know, however, that the advice concerning wheat bran was incorrect, as it can, in fact, exacerbate rather than reduce abdominal pain and does not always help constipation.

A long-term lowering of fibre intake is not ideal as it reduces dietary variety and may result in nutritional deficiencies. Fibre is important in bulking and softening stools; it also benefits the microbiome, so it is vital to include fibre that is tolerated. Experts suggest around 30 g daily is needed, but this level may not be tolerated by all with IBS. High levels might not always be useful in those with a very sluggish bowel.

If you're increasing fibre intake, perhaps for constipation, do so gradually. Golden or milled linseeds can be effective in improving stool function and can also help with bloating. Try them in porridge, yogurt or a salad, and take with water. Work up to a maximum of four tablespoons a day, and give yourself up to six months for your bowel to adjust.

Ispaghula husk (such as Fybogel) can be tried as a laxative source of soluble fibre.

Microbial treatments

Our 'good' gut bacteria help keep our guts – and indeed our bodies – healthy in many ways, but we know that levels can be reduced in those with IBS. Can we do anything to help boost their numbers?

Fermented foods

Live yogurt, kefir (fermented milk), sauerkraut (pickled cabbage), kimchi (pickled fermented vegetables), tempeh (fermented soya), filmjolk (Scandinavian soured milk), miso (fermented soya seasoning) and raw vinegar are high in probiotic bacteria, and can add variety to the diet.

Probiotics

Can a supplemental probiotic help boost our good bacteria? This is a very attractive concept and there is a plethora of products on the market aimed at doing just that.

Probiotic supplements have been found to be effective overall, but evidence is weak for individual products and for some there is none at all – making it hard for healthcare practitioners to know which products to recommend. Not only is there variation among people, their symptoms and their microbiome, there is also variety in the products in terms of dose, bacterial strains, species and mixture of bacteria, the dosage form (capsule or liquid), the carrier (yogurt, fruit juice, fermented barley), the shelf life of live products and whether or not the bacteria survive their passage through the stomach.

There is no risk from probiotics – unless you are receiving immunosuppressant treatment, in which case they should not be used – and healthcare practitioners suggest that trials of any one product should be undertaken for at least one month in the dose and method advised by the manufacturer, while symptoms are monitored. If you find the product effective, you should continue to take it; if not, you could try another product. Be aware that not all your symptoms may improve with probiotics and their effects may be minor, and consider the costs of the product and if it contains FODMAP sources. Some people find they work; others don't. However, probiotics are worth considering as a first-line treatment.

As research is active and continuing in this area, check Julie's Blog for up-to-date information about which probiotic may prove useful for which IBS symptom, as we learn more (<www.clinicalalimentary.wordpress.com>).

Fluid intake

Many people do not drink sufficient fluids: the average person needs six to eight glasses per day. If you have IBS with constipation you could supplement the usual six glasses with up to six more, to see if this improves your symptoms. If you have diarrhoea you might need more too. The best sources are water and dilutable squash (choose 'no added sugar' versions, without polyol sweeteners such as sorbitol, mannitol, maltitol, xylitol and isomalt), although tea can be consumed as the caffeine content of tea is low, be it black, green or white. That said, very occasionally tea can cause constipation, so it's worth reducing consumption to see if this improves. Peppermint tea is fine.

Your urine should be pale yellow; dark yellow or orange means you should drink more. Discuss symptoms with your doctor if you have been advised to limit fluid intake because of a medical condition.

Carbonated drinks

Most of the gas present in fizzy drinks is expelled from the stomach by belching, but inevitably some travels down into the large bowel to form gas and this doesn't help symptoms.

Chewing gum

This may aggravate symptoms of IBS as chewing gum can increase the quantity of air you swallow – those with bloating, beware. Some are sensitive to polyol sweeteners such as sorbitol, which are contained in much sugar-free gum.

The way we eat

Food maintains life, and consuming it is meant to be pleasurable. Yet some who have IBS have a love–hate relationship with food, due to the symptoms that eating can provoke. But this may not only or necessarily be due to the *type* of food eaten – but the *manner* in which it is eaten. Mindful eating is recommended. Here are some tips that may help:

- At work, don't eat at your desk. Get out of the office.
- Don't eat on the move. Sit at a table. It will help posture, which may help digestion.
- Slow down. Be more aware that you are eating – chew each mouthful well (around 15 times is ideal) and enjoy the taste. If it helps, put your sandwich or your knife and fork down between mouthfuls.

- Eat in company, to slow yourself down. Keep conversation neutral – no topics that may lead to arguments or stress, as this can increase adrenaline levels, which suppress digestion. Talk about the food!
- Don't overeat. It takes 20 minutes for your brain to register that you have begun eating, and 15 minutes for it to know you are full. Rushing increases the likelihood you'll become uncomfortably full and susceptible to symptoms.
- Avoid swallowing air. It's natural to swallow some air as you eat – and belching at the end of a meal can help release some of it – but fast eating or speaking with your mouth full can mean you end up swallowing excessive amounts, which can travel down to the bowel and lead to wind. (Ill-fitting dentures may result in air swallowing when you eat, so see your dentist if this may be a problem.)
- Eat regularly. Skipping meals can result in symptoms, so have three meals a day with no more than five hours between meals. If you are underweight, snacks between meals are fine.

4

Identifying triggers

Although making minor healthy eating changes and taking dietary advice from your GP can improve matters for some with mild IBS, for others there could be a deeper dietary problem or trigger to identify – and those with moderate to severe IBS may need particularly specialist advice from a dietitian.

What is a dietitian?

A dietitian is a trained professional who is qualified in the science of nutrition and can translate that knowledge and expertise into personalized, practical dietary advice and guidance for those who need it most.

Dietitians work in many areas, including the NHS, the food industry, education, occupational health, government departments and private healthcare.

The job title 'dietitian' is legally protected: it can only be used by those registered with the Health and Care Professions Council (HCPC), a body that regulates practitioners and ensures they meet certain stringent standards. Dietitians are the *only* professionals with the training to treat people with complex medical conditions where nutrition is part of the treatment, such as IBS.

The job title 'nutritionist' is not legally protected and can be used electively. However, the Association of Nutritionists is a body for those who have a recognized degree in nutrition and meet strict standards. Registered nutritionists provide healthy eating advice to those without disease.

Below degree-level qualifications in nutrition – such as in so-called nutritional therapy – are offered by bodies such as the Institute of Optimum Nutrition, but job titles such as 'nutritional therapist' or, indeed, 'diet expert' are not independently regulated. Such practitioners may use non-evidence-based methods of diagnosis or treatment, including supplementation, so-called detoxing and perhaps unnecessary dietary restrictions on the basis of unvalidated tests.

Unfortunately, dietitians have something of a reputation of being the 'diet police' in some quarters, but this couldn't be further from the truth. A dietitian will work holistically with you and your lifestyle to help you develop a plan that is achievable. The treatment that is provided will be given with discussion and agreement with you. There will be no finger-wagging!

The first appointment

Before you attend, write down any questions you have. Time will go quickly, you may be provided with a great deal of information and otherwise you may forget what you wanted to ask. Ground covered will include topics such as:

- your symptom history;
- the tests that preceded your IBS diagnosis;
- medication you have tried or are still taking;
- any dietary exclusion or manipulation you have tried;
- your current food and drink intake, both during a typical day, and over the course of the week;
- family history of bowel or allergic disorders.

Is food making you ill?

Many wonder this and it is a question your dietitian is equipped to help you answer.

Is it a food allergy?

This is a common concern among people with IBS, but the vast majority will *not* have a food allergy. Confusion can arise as the term is misused by many lay people and some alternative therapists to mean any kind of undesirable reaction or response to food.

A food allergy is a very specific physical reaction, due to an abnormal response by our immune system – the collection of cells responsible for 'defence' and protecting the body against infection.

The most common is a type I reaction, affecting around 2 per cent of the population and typically caused by a protein component in foods such as nuts, peanuts, eggs, fish, milk or sesame.

Symptoms, which may be triggered by even a tiny trace of the culprit food and occur very quickly after consumption, can include oral swelling, asthma, nettle rash, swelling of body tissues (angio-oedema) and anaphylaxis (breathing difficulties, light-headedness and feeling faint or collapsing). Abdominal symptoms of nausea, vomiting, abdominal pain and diarrhoea are also possible, however, meaning that very occasionally a food allergy may be misinterpreted as IBS.

A 'milder' form, more common in people with hay fever, is called oral allergy syndrome or pollen allergy syndrome. This is typically caused by raw fruit and raw vegetables, and results in symptoms localized to the mouth, such as itchy or swelling lips, tongue, throat or gums.

Blood tests are available for type I food allergy (except oral allergy syndrome), but they are not sufficiently accurate in themselves and other investigations may be required. These can include skin-prick tests (where foods are 'scratched' into the skin and any local reaction measured), plus a clinical history and a food challenge.

If you have a confirmed food allergy or are concerned a food allergy diagnosis has been missed, mention it to your dietitian. If a food allergy is suspected and the culprit is unknown, your GP should refer you to an immunologist.

Type IV allergy

This also involves the immune system but is slower – with symptoms occurring up to 48 hours after exposure to the food. These may occasionally include dermatitis or eczema, but many are bowel-based symptoms that mimic those in IBS and food intolerance, making diagnosis a real challenge for practitioners – especially since there is no blood test for this type of food allergy.

In practice, it may be diagnosed – via an elimination diet (see page 41) – as a food intolerance, although if you have a history of eczema, asthma or hay fever, a specialist dietitian may suspect a type IV food allergy under certain circumstances.

However, this allergy is rare, and for the vast majority of those with IBS, any existing reaction to food is likely to be a food intolerance.

Is it a food intolerance?

A food intolerance is an adverse reaction to a food in which the immune system is not involved.

Most food intolerances are a reaction to a sugar or carbohydrate component of food, perhaps due to the absence or low levels of a digestive enzyme – such as the lack of lactase, which causes the symptoms of lactose intolerance.

Unlike people with food allergies, where a tiny amount of a trigger food can bring on symptoms, individuals with food intolerances can often tolerate small or modest amounts of an offending food, and working with a dietitian can help you to identify both your trigger foods and to some extent what quantities of them that, if ingested, will mean you will react adversely to those foods so you then know what your limits are.

How will a dietitian do that? The answer lies in the elimination diet.

Elimination diets

An elimination diet is a diagnostic diet that works by eliminating certain foods from the diet in the short term to see if symptoms improve; if they do improve, those foods are gradually and individually reintroduced into the diet to monitor whether or not there are any responses to them and identify possible tolerance levels.

This is considered the 'gold standard' method of identifying food intolerances, but the elimination diet can be restrictive and challenging. It should, therefore, only be undertaken for a short period of time in order to ensure that the diet will not be nutritionally compromised.

Historically, an elimination diet has been used for IBS, but in recent years our understanding of food intolerances in the condition has improved considerably and the low-FODMAP diet – which is, in essence, a partial elimination diet – is likely to be the front-line approach your dietitian suggests.

The low-FODMAP diet

'FODMAP' is an acronym. It stands for 'Fermentable Oligosaccharides, Disaccharides, Monosaccharides And Polyols'.

'Oligosaccharides', 'disaccharides', 'monosaccharides' and 'polyols' are four complicated-sounding terms for four groups of simple sugars or carbohydrates, all of which occur naturally in plant and dairy foods to varying degrees.

In general, these sugars are poorly absorbed and poorly digested in the small intestine. As they pass through, they draw water into the bowel, then as they pass further into the large intestine, they are fermented by the healthy bacteria present there, leading to gas production. These are perfectly normal processes in all of us.

Some individuals' digestive systems are better equipped to handle them than those of others, however, such as those with low levels of key digestive enzymes or whose guts are particularly ineffective at absorbing two particular sugars, lactose and fructose. If too great a level of FODMAPs reaches the large intestine, water can be drawn in and excess gas may be produced, leading to sometimes severe symptoms of bloating, wind and diarrhoea. Some of these can be amplified in those with IBS.

The low-FODMAP diet was developed by a team of researchers from Monash University in Australia. Research shows that it offers

Getting to see a FODMAP-trained dietitian

The National Institute for Health and Care Excellence (NICE) states that anyone requiring treatment with a low-FODMAP diet should have access to a trained practitioner. Currently, only dietitians have received this training. In the UK, mentioning these guidelines can help to support your attempts to get a referral if you are struggling.

Increasing numbers of NHS departments are offering group education schemes and some hospital dietetic departments offer their own version of the low-FODMAP diet, so do enquire locally.

You can also find dietitians privately. The British Dietetic Association and King's College London (KCL) hold lists of FODMAP-trained dietitians. Some offer private consultations via Skype, which can help if you are in a remote area (see the Useful addresses section for links).

benefits for around 70 per cent of those with IBS, but only in those supported throughout by a FODMAP-trained dietitian. It is vital you do likewise, as the diet is complex and should not be undertaken lightly. The temptation to go it alone may be strong – especially if you are impatient for a solution – but failure is far more likely if you attempt it without professional support, which may put you off trying again in future.

What is involved?

The diet itself begins with an elimination (or restriction) of all high-FODMAP foods for four to eight weeks.

This is followed by a reintroduction in stages – where foods are individually reincorporated into the diet, each over the course of three days, in increasing quantities – to identify intolerances of, and personal threshold tolerance levels for, various foods.

Tolerance levels vary considerably between individuals with IBS and many foods may be tolerated at everyday levels.

A useful analogy is to consider a cup as your personal 'FODMAP container'. If you eat too many FODMAP-containing foods, you may get a spillage of contents – that is, symptoms. Everyone's cup size is different – and the low-FODMAP elimination diet will help you to identify the size of yours.

High- and low-FODMAP foods

The list in Table 4.1 (overleaf) is by no means exhaustive but shows you some of the more common foods that are permitted and excluded during the elimination phase.

As a relatively young field, research into FODMAP content of food is continuing, and up-to-date accurate information will be available from your dietitian. Do not trust data about FODMAP content online unless it comes from a reputable source, such as Monash University in Australia, King's College London or a FODMAP-trained dietitian.

FODMAP types

It is useful to consider the types of FODMAPs in more detail, since not all may be problematic. Even those that are may be tolerable at reduced levels.

Table 4.1 High- and low-FODMAP foods

Food type	High-FODMAP foods	Low-FODMAP foods
Grain/starchy carbohydrates	Wheat (all types, including bulgar, couscous, freekeh, spelt), barley, rye; all flour, pasta or noodles, bread,* cereal products, and other baked products from these grains, including pastries, cakes, biscuits and crackers (* unless 100 per cent sourdough spelt bread)	Rice (all types), potato, oats, buckwheat, quinoa; gluten-free flour, bread, pasta or noodles, savoury crackers and unsweetened cereals made from these grains; 100 per cent sourdough spelt bread; polenta
Protein	Beans and pulses – lentils, chickpeas, beans, split peas, tofu (silken)	All meat, all fish and seafood, tofu (firm), egg, Quorn (but check for wheat, onion and garlic)
Fruit	Apple, pear, watermelon, Sharon fruit or persimmon, blackberries, figs, stone-containing fruits (apricot, date, peach, plum or prune, cherry), mango, tinned fruit in apple or pear juice	Banana, rhubarb, melon (cantaloupe and honeydew), blueberries, raspberries, strawberries, cranberries, kiwi, papaya, passion fruit, pineapple, grapes and all citrus fruits
Vegetables	Onion (all types), garlic, mushroom, Jerusalem artichoke, cauliflower, celery, beetroot, asparagus, sugar-snap peas	Lettuces, cabbage, carrot, celeriac, chard, chicory, courgette, aubergine, beansprouts, green beans, kale, cucumber, pumpkin, radish, parsnip, bell peppers, spinach, swede, tomato, turnip
Dairy	Milk (whole, semi-skimmed, skimmed, powdered, condensed); yogurt (whole, low-fat and drinking); processed cheese, cottage cheese, reduced-fat Cheddar, cream cheese, halloumi, ricotta, quark, low-fat soft cheese	Reduced-lactose milk and cheese. Butter, mature or hard cheeses such as full fat Cheddar, Parmesan, Edam, feta (see pages 75–6 for vegan alternatives)

Food type	High-FODMAP foods	Low-FODMAP foods
Nuts and seeds	Cashews, pistachios, sesame, tahini, hummus	Walnuts, pumpkin seeds
Condiments and savoury flavourings	Chutney, HP Sauce; check all condiments for added onion and garlic	Salt (use sparingly), pepper, vinegar, Worcestershire sauce, garlic-infused oil, capers, miso paste, peanut butter, mustard, soy sauce, Marmite, Sarson's Browning
Sugar, sweeteners, confectionery	Honey, agave nectar, fructose syrups, polyols (sorbitol, mannitol, xylitol, isomalt)	Table sugar, glucose, golden syrup, dark chocolate, jam, marmalade (made with low-FODMAP fruit). 100 per cent maple syrup; artificial sweeteners (stevia, aspartame, acesulfame K, saccharin, sucralose)
Beverages	Camomile tea, fennel tea	Tea, peppermint tea, coffee

Fructose

Fructose is a monosaccharide – a single sugar unit – that occurs naturally in fruit and is commonly found in sweet sugar syrups, such as corn syrup and glucose-fructose syrup.

Excessive intake of fructose can lead to symptoms in most individuals, as it is not well absorbed. Almost half of us poorly absorb 25 g of fructose (found in two wedges of watermelon, or 2½ tablespoons of honey or 80 g of dates, for example), so fructose intolerance should be considered a strong suspect in symptoms of IBS. In fact, it is more common than lactose intolerance, although it remains under-recognized in the medical community. One study found that three-quarters of those with IBS and fructose malabsorption experienced symptomatic relief from a fructose-modified diet.

Fructose is also found in sucrose – better known as table sugar – where it is bound with glucose. However, in this form it is more actively absorbed by the body, so table sugar is not considered a FODMAP. That said, no more than 5 per cent of our energy intake (roughly 100 calories) should come from such added sugar.

Lactose

Lactose is a disaccharide sugar – consisting of two single sugar units, glucose and galactose – found naturally in the milk of all mammals.

The lining of our small bowel secretes an enzyme, lactase, that breaks down lactose, but production of this enzyme can be scaled down as we age, or temporarily halted because of a gastrointestinal infection. Lactose that is not broken down can ferment and can trigger unpleasant symptoms, such as frothy diarrhoea.

Although in rare cases lactose intolerance can be present from early childhood (primary lactose intolerance), it more commonly develops in later life (secondary lactose intolerance), especially in certain ethnic groups, such as Asian, African or South American.

In recent years, products have been developed that are 'pre-digested' with lactase, and these low-lactose or lactose-free milks, yogurts and cheeses can be useful during the elimination stage to help maintain calcium intake. However, most hard cheeses – especially mature and full fat cheeses – are low in lactose anyway, so your dietitian may suggest that alternatives are unnecessary.

Secondary lactose intolerance can occur in IBS and also after a gastrointestinal infection or gastroenteritis. This can be temporary, and removal of lactose from the diet need not be lifelong – this is why it is important to gradually reincorporate lactose into your diet following an episode of food poisoning to see if the intolerance has resolved.

Lactose-free cow's milk has the advantage of containing similar levels of calcium to standard cow's milk. Any choice of alternative milks should be fortified with calcium and vitamin D (vitamin D helps absorption of calcium). Remember that the low-FODMAP diet is not a milk-free diet; lactose-free milk has nutritional benefits over some animal milk alternatives. Lactose can also be found in some medications, but usually at a tolerably small dose. A pharmacist can identify medications without lactose if need be.

Oligosaccharides

'Oligo' means 'a few', indicating that oligosaccharides are formed from several or a number of chains of sugar units. They include fructans (or sometimes fructo-oligosaccharides – FOS) and galactans (or sometimes galacto-oligosaccharides – GOS).

Raffinose, stachyose and verbascose are types of GOS found in pulses and legumes – that is, chickpeas, lentils, all types of beans, and peas. They are poorly absorbed by everyone, but only cause negative reactions for people with IBS. They are responsible for beans' windy reputation!

Fructans are found in wheat, onion, garlic, artichokes and chicory and can be added to foods as prebiotics, to promote a healthy bowel.

Polyols

Sometimes called the sugar alcohols but not alcoholic in any sense, the polyols include sorbitol, mannitol, xylitol, lactitol and isomalt.

Sorbitol is found in some fruits and vegetables and in sugar-free confectionery, for example. Food products warning of potential laxative effects with over-consumption usually signify the presence of a polyol.

Is it always carbohydrates that are fermented?

Recent studies have shown that red meat can also be fermented by bacteria in the bowel, if large amounts are consumed. Beef, lamb, pork, veal, venison and goat are good sources of iron, protein, B vitamins and zinc, and should be included in the diet two to three times a week if you have no ethical or cultural reasons to avoid them. A suitable portion size is 70 g. Eating much more can increase the risk of bowel cancer in the long term and may elicit symptoms of IBS for some. Try switching *some* of your red meat portions to alternatives such as chicken and turkey if you do eat more than three portions a week.

The elimination phase

During your first appointment, your dietitian will give you information on how to follow the low-FODMAP diet and change particular meals. That time with your dietitian will go quickly, leaving you little opportunity to contemplate your new diet. This usually comes afterwards, when you are at home, armed with all the information.

There is a saying that if something doesn't challenge you, it won't change you – in other words, you have to step outside your normal eating and change your diet to improve your symptoms. This can be particularly the case if some of the foods you are going to eat are not part of your typical diet.

The best advice is to carefully read the information and plan your eating and shopping before you start. This is your challenge, and effort is needed to see improvement in all aspects of life. Taking time to prepare is better than diving into the diet immediately and ending up feeling restricted and hungry.

A dietitian is unlikely to provide complete food plans for you, as they rarely work and most people don't follow them well. Planning your diet around your own likes and dislikes will make it easier for you to stick to.

Remember: the diet is not for ever, but for two months *maximum*. Contemplating the consequences of eating high-FODMAP food may be all you need to keep on track. You do not have to keep a food diary during this phase but it may help.

Nutritional consequences

Aim to include as much variety as possible to ensure the nutrition your body needs.

The diet can be low in calcium and fibre (and possibly iron in those who do not eat meat). To counteract this, consume low-lactose dairy products, wholegrain wheat-free starchy carbohydrates or fortified breakfast cereals, and five portions of low-FODMAP fruit and vegetables. Portion sizes of low-FODMAP fruit (80 g), fruit juice (100 ml) and dried fruit (13 g) are limited, but low-FODMAP vegetables are not. One or two high-FODMAP foods are permitted in small amounts – your dietitian can advise on portion sizes.

Vegans can consume a small amount of rinsed canned pulses (two tablespoons), which can increase variety and nutritional quality.

Probiotics might be useful at this time if your dietitian advises you to try them (see page 35). However, as the diet is only for a two-month period, reduction in bacterial profile is unlikely to have long-term consequences as long as the reintroductions are completed, and some prebiotic foods can be consumed. Plus, if you take a probiotic alongside the low-FODMAP diet you might not know which of these two changes have been effective.

Meal ideas

Here are some suggestions. See Chapter 6 for more and Appendix 2 for recipes.

Breakfast

- Porridge made with lactose-free milk topped with strawberries
- Gluten-free toast and peanut butter
- Gluten-free muffin or crumpet (see Appendix 2) with poached egg
- Gluten-free pancakes with a drizzle of maple syrup and plain lactose-free yogurt
- Gluten-free bread dipped in beaten egg (French toast – see Appendix 2) topped with chopped low-FODMAP fruit
- Home-made muesli with lactose-free yogurt.

Lunch

- Chicken or fish salad with lettuce, cucumber, rocket, peppers
- Rice or corn cakes with ham
- Gluten-free wrap served with ham or cheese and green leaves
- Jacket potato with tuna and light mayonnaise
- Cheese soufflé (see Appendix 2)
- Pumpkin soup (see Appendix 2) or other soup with low-FODMAP ingredients
- Rice salad (home-made)
- Pasta salad (home-made with gluten- or wheat-free pasta)
- Home-made gluten-free sandwiches.

Evening meals

- Tuna pasta bake (made with wheat-free pasta)
- Chicken breast with boiled potatoes and carrots
- Grilled fish with boiled rice and roasted peppers
- Stuffed aubergines (see Appendix 2) with green salad
- Fish cakes (see Appendix 2) with roasted low-FODMAP vegetables
- Thai pork loin (see Appendix 2) with boiled rice and pak choi
- Turkey burgers on gluten-free muffin (see Appendix 2).

Desserts

- One portion of low-FODMAP fruit
- Lactose-free yogurt
- Jelly and lactose-free ice-cream
- Rice pudding made with lactose-free milk.

When will I feel better?

Some people feel better quickly – within two to three weeks. Most, however, will be feeling better by six to eight weeks.

If you do not feel better in two months, then contact your dietitian as it may be that you have inadvertently included a FODMAP food in your diet. You might be asked to complete a food and symptom diary to identify whether or not you are eating a FODMAP or to check if other foods are causing your symptoms.

If you have followed the low-FODMAP diet, using up-to-date information from a reputable source and with dietetic help, but have not experienced any improvement, you should reintroduce eliminated foods and consider alternative treatments.

If you are still experiencing diarrhoea, it could be NCGS and a gluten-free diet may be needed (see page 57). Identifying this could be tricky, but one possibility is to complete a gluten-free low-FODMAP diet and reintroduce sourdough spelt bread, which is believed to be tolerated by those intolerant to FODMAPs but contains gluten. If symptoms result, then NCGS might be the cause, although, again, the use of this as a diagnostic tool is not fully established or researched.

The low-FODMAP diet and constipation

Can the low-FODMAP approach work for IBS-C as well as IBS-D?

Studies in IBS-C patients show the diet is not *always* effective for slow bowel transit – in other words, it does not resolve constipation for everyone – but *can* be useful in improving other IBS-C symptoms. Clinical experience suggests that the diet works for some, but not others.

One possible reason for this is that the low-FODMAP diet can increase the amount of fibre consumed, compared to a previously low level of consumption that was perhaps contributing to constipation for some people with IBS-C.

Another possibility is that the diet reduces fibre intake for some people – again useful if the constipation is caused by a very slow-moving bowel where high fibre intakes are sometimes unhelpful. More research is needed to identify when the diet is beneficial for IBS-C.

If you have had long-standing constipation and many treatments have been tried, along with general lifestyle advice to include plenty of sources of fibre and fluid in your diet, all without success, your dietitian may not advise the low-FODMAP diet.

The diet is likely to be given with particular emphasis on increasing your fibre and fluid intake too, if your dietitian finds these are low. The low-FODMAP diet can be lower in fibre than a general healthy diet, so it is important to address this aspect as required.

If you have tried both the low-FODMAP diet and the low-FODMAP diet with increased fibre sources and have had no symptom improvement, then dietary treatment is unlikely to be helpful for you. This is not unusual, as 30 per cent experience no improvement. (Biofeedback training – see page 26 – may help in this situation.)

What fluids and fibre are suitable?

Trial high-fibre gluten-free cereals or wholegrain sourdough spelt bread. Ensure you check the amount of fibre on the label – just because a gluten-free bread is brown doesn't guarantee it is high in fibre (caramel or molasses are often used to impart colour).

Some gluten-free foods contain a fibre called psyllium husk flour – this is used in bread to act as a humectant, meaning it retains water, to keep the bread moist. Psyllium does the same thing in the bowel, increasing stool bulk and keeping stools soft. The laxative version, psyllium husk, has been anecdotally reported to increase gas and bloating but has not been FODMAP-tested. Most people *do* tolerate gluten-free bread and you should include it, but try to vary your carbohydrate sources too. Aim for 30 g fibre daily. Try rice bran or wholegrain rice for additional fibre. Have no more than three portions of fruit a day, and include permitted vegetables to bring this figure up to at least five fruit and vegetable portions per day.

If you have previously severely restricted the amount of fibre in your diet, it is best to increase your intake slowly, so your bowel can adjust. Here is an example of how you might do this.

Week 1   Introduce low-FODMAP fruit and vegetables by one portion (80 g fresh or 13 g dried fruit) per day until you consume your recommended five a day (maximum three portions of fruit).

Week 2   Introduce wholegrain carbohydrates (brown rice, rice bran, oats and fibre and seeded wheat-free breads) by one portion (one slice of bread or 30 g oats) per day during the week until three portions per day have been achieved.

Week 3   Include a small handful of nuts and seeds.

If your doctor has advised you to take a laxative, continue with this throughout, unless you have persistent loose stools. Plus, certain laxatives can be good to use alongside the low-FODMAP diet if constipation is a problem (the exception here is lactulose, which is a high-FODMAP product).

Reflux and IBS

If you have reflux, the general lifestyle advice can include to avoid 'acidic' and spicy foods.

If you have previously stopped eating citrus fruits as a result, you should try to reincorporate them; some find they can eat them because they are low-FODMAP foods and reflux symptoms can improve when following the diet (although the diet is not advisable for reflux if you have *not* been diagnosed with IBS).

Spicy meals might include garlic and onion, so it again may be worth trying some recipes for foods that include chilli but no onion or garlic, to see if you can include small amounts.

The best time to reintroduce any previously excluded foods that are low FODMAP is while following the elimination phase, once you have had an improvement in symptoms.

Reintroduction

When your symptoms have improved substantially or fully, individual reintroductions can begin.

This part is important. Here, you will identify intolerances and be able to 'relax' the diet to enjoy some of the foods you have excluded. It will also allow you to include some of the prebiotic foods that are beneficial to gut bacteria.

There is no standard order: you are free to decide which FODMAP to reintroduce and when – perhaps starting with foods you have missed most.

As with all aspects of identifying food intolerances, planning reintroductions will help you.

The tested food is increased by portion in one meal over three days – you should use the same food item for each of the days.

If you do not tolerate Day 1's introduction, add the food and portion size to your 'FODMAPs to avoid' list of foods.

If Day 1 is tolerated, progress to Day 2. If not tolerated, add the food and Day 1 portion size to your 'permitted' list and Day 2 portion size to your 'food to avoid' list.

If tolerated, progress to Day 3, and if the food does not trigger symptoms it can be added to your list of 'safe' foods – although you should not start to consume it while you are completing the FODMAP reintroductions. This is because a stable baseline low-FODMAP level needs to be maintained to enable you to identify FODMAP tolerance levels effectively. If you were to start adding large amounts of tolerated FODMAPs at once, you might experience symptoms through consuming too many in one meal.

This means the low-FODMAP diet should be followed while each FODMAP introduction is undertaken. It is important to have three symptom-free days before each reintroduction.

If you experience symptoms, exclude the food and wait for symptoms to resolve before reintroducing any new foods (usually, three days is enough).

Record the amounts of foods you can and can't tolerate. This will help in future if you inadvertently relax the diet and find symptoms increase.

If you've had symptoms for some time and these have improved significantly you may be worried about the reintroductions. If so, discuss it with your dietitian, as portion sizes can be adjusted to help reduce your anxiety. You *will* have some symptoms during the process but they are unlikely to be as severe as before. That said, prepare for it: complete reintroductions when having symptoms is more 'convenient' (for example, when you can be at home) and have medications to hand. The symptoms will be short-lived and will *not* be harmful in the long term.

If you find you can't reintroduce any foods without symptoms, tell your dietitian, and do likewise if you have particularly high levels of anxiety. The advice in Chapter 7 may also help.

Example reintroductions

In order to reintroduce disaccharides, monosaccharides and the oligosaccharide galacto-oligosaccharides (GOS), you only need to introduce one food, such as milk for the disaccharide lactose, honey for the monosaccharide fructose and beans for the GOS.

- **Lactose** a small (125 ml) glass of milk on Day 1, two glasses on Day 2 and three glasses on Day 3. (NB: some sources suggest yogurt can be used in place of milk, but as the lactose content of yogurt varies, milk may be better. It can be spread through the day.)
- **Fructose** one teaspoon of honey on Day 1, two teaspoons on Day 2, and three on Day 3.
- **GOS** one tablespoon of beans on Day 1, two tablepoons on Day 2 and three on Day 3.
- **Polyol sorbitol** three tablespoons of broccoli on Day 1, six on Day 2 and nine on Day 3.
- **Polyol mannitol** two tablespoons of cauliflower on Day 1, four on Day 2 and six on Day 3.

Fructans and FOS are a little more complicated – onion, garlic and wheat should be introduced individually.

- **Fructans wheat** one slice of bread on Day 1, two slices on Day 2 and three on Day 3.
- **Fructans onion** one tablespoon on Day 1, two tablespoons on Day 2 and three on Day 3.
- **Fructans garlic** quarter of a clove of garlic on Day 1, ½ on Day 2 and a full clove on Day 3 – this can be raw or cooked.

Some people may successfully introduce the 'easier' FODMAPs – lactose, fructose and GOS, which can be identified with one food – and then have a bit of a 'break' from the diet and follow a tolerated diet for a while before reintroducing the more challenging FODMAPs, such as fructans. If you do this, when you recommence reintroductions you must go back on the low-FODMAP diet, to ensure the stable baseline. Bear in mind that the full reintroduction should take around two months, in total.

Any food containing more than one FODMAP type should also be introduced individually. Examples include watermelon (fructans, mannitol and fructose) and mushrooms (fructans and mannitol).

When you have tested most foods by this one-by-one method of reintroduction, experiment cautiously with having more than one reintroduced tolerated food and carefully monitoring your symptoms. Remember that your FODMAP 'cup' may overflow if you consume a large amount of different FODMAP types in one meal.

There is no need to introduce foods that you are never likely to eat.

5

Diets for IBS

With the help of your GP and/or your dietitian, you may by now have identified any triggers that set off your symptoms and your healthcare providers may have recommended some changes to your diet. These may be minor or they may be more considerable, requiring you to follow a more structured, carefully designed diet.

In the next chapter, we look at issues surrounding shopping for food, labelling and eating out, but in this chapter we examine some of the diets in more detail and advise on safe foods, cooking and nutrition.

The modified low-FODMAP diet

There is no 'one size fits all' modified low-FODMAP diet, so it is impossible to give detailed information about diet and nutrition here.

Assuming you have carefully undertaken the elimination and reintroduction protocol described in the previous chapter, this modified low-FODMAP diet is the third and final phase of the low-FODMAP diet plan – and will be the one that is suitable for *you* personally.

It includes high-FODMAP foods, consumed at levels that don't result in symptoms for you, and of course low-FODMAP foods.

Knowing your particular triggers is important. Keep a list of foods that you can eat pinned up as a reminder. Try not to get into a rut with your diet, eating the same foods every day.

It's also important, where possible, to consume high-FODMAP foods that come with particular nutritional benefits – but only to the point of tolerance. For instance, the fructans in wheat, onion, garlic, artichokes and chicory act as a prebiotic to promote healthy bowel bacteria. If you can manage small amounts, consume them.

Recipes, books and appropriate websites (see the Useful addresses section) can give you further ideas if you're struggling, and there'll be more pointers in the next chapter too.

The gluten-free diet (GFD)

This must be followed strictly if you have coeliac disease (CD) and is advised if you have non-coeliac gluten sensitivity (NCGS) – although in this second case we don't know the degree to which small quantities of gluten can be tolerated, if at all. What if you don't have such a diagnosis?

Occasionally, a GFD may be advised if you have neurological symptoms (such as difficulties with your balance and walking) and digestive symptoms or a very strong family history of CD along with your IBS diagnosis.

It may also be trialled if a low-FODMAP plan has failed to resolve chronic diarrhoea.

A GFD should only be undertaken with the support of your dietitian, and not experimentally on your own volition, as it can affect future tests and your nutritional status.

What is a GFD?

A GFD is simply a diet that excludes the following gluten-containing grains:

- wheat
- barley
- rye
- oats (unless labelled gluten-free).

It also excludes:

- all varieties or hybrids of these grains (such as durum, einkorn, emmer, KAMUT® and other khorasan wheat, spelt, triticale);
- most forms of wheat (bran, bulgur, couscous, freekeh, rusk, semolina, wheat protein, wheat starch, wheatgerm, for example).

So the GFD must exclude all products containing the grains listed above and all products containing ingredients derived from them – with only a few exceptions.

It includes all fruit, vegetables, nuts, seeds, non-gluten grains, meats, fish, natural dairy products and eggs, and products and ingredients derived only from these foods.

The wheat issue

Although there are several grains you need to avoid, it is wheat that you'll encounter most regularly. It is widespread in the Western diet, partly because flour-based products such as breads and pastas are staples, and partly because of wheat's additional role as a stabilizer, thickener or 'filler' in processed foods. It may also be used to 'dust' products and prevent them clumping together, and can turn up in surprising places.

Wheat-based or wheat-containing products may include:

- most flours, breads and baked products – both sweet and savoury;
- many cereals;
- most pastas, some noodles;
- some meat and fish products – burgers, pies, sausages, pâtés and battered products such as fish fingers;
- some vegetarian products – battered vegetables, pâtés, some tinned soups;
- some plant milks;
- some dairy products, such as cheese spreads, thickened milks and creams;
- confectionery, including chocolate bars, cereal bars, sweets, chewing gum and liquorice;
- stock cubes, gravy granules, condiments and blended seasonings.

Dairy- or milk-free diet

The low-FODMAP diet is not a milk-free diet, and for the vast majority of people with IBS eliminating milk is unnecessary.

If you were diagnosed with a milk protein allergy as a child, were later told you had grown out of the allergy but have since been diagnosed with IBS, it may be worth alerting your dietitian to this, as a milk-free diet may potentially improve symptoms. This *should not* be attempted without advice as some people can have rare extreme allergic reactions if milk is excluded and they are later exposed to trace milk contamination in the diet.

However, if you are vegan or have an 'active' milk protein allergy, you will have to be milk-free. If you are also following a low-FODMAP diet, ensure replacement milks are fortified with calcium and vitamin D. See Chapter 6 for vegan alternatives to milk. Milk is found in processed foods and food labels have to be checked – see Chapter 6 for further advice.

Note that 'dairy-free' means 'cow's milk-free' and 'milk-free' means 'animal milk-free'. All animal milks contain the FODMAP lactose, and if you have an allergy to cow's milk you are likely to have an allergy to the milk of goats and sheep too.

Vegan diets

A vegan diet is free of all animal products, including eggs and honey, and can be healthy if care is taken to ensure it is nutritionally complete and not too high in calories.

Some struggle to follow a vegan low-FODMAP diet as beans and pulses are excluded during the elimination phase because of their GOS content. Quinoa is an excellent source of protein, containing all essential amino acids; peanut butter is good too.

To ensure adequate iron in your diet include some dark green leafy vegetables (kale, pak choi, chard and spinach are reasonable sources) or sesame seeds, taken with a small (100 ml) amount of orange or other citrus juice (the vitamin C helps the uptake of iron in the body). Fortified breakfast cereals may also help and contain B vitamins – have them with fortified vegan milks.

The trick to a strong vegan diet is variety and including tolerated amounts of FODMAP-containing foods. For example, include small amounts of rinsed canned lentils or chickpeas for both protein and extra iron. Small amounts of seeds and permitted nuts, including up to two Brazil nuts for the mineral selenium, are good; flaxseed, walnuts or rapeseed oil are good sources of omega-3 fatty acids. For iodine, use iodized salt or try nori (seaweed).

Supplementing your IBS diet

Whether you're on a modified FODMAP diet, a milk-free diet, a gluten-free diet and/or a vegan diet, other than modifying your food and drink intake what else can you take to help?

Some with IBS come to follow a heavily restricted diet, and this can lead to long-term vitamin and mineral deficiencies. Supplements should only be considered under the guidance of a doctor or dietitian, when blood tests show low levels or diet analyses suggest low intake.

Always read the label of supplements – not only for directions of use and dosage, but to check ingredients if you have food allergies or coeliac disease, as some may contain FODMAPs, allergens or gluten.

Vitamins

Those following a varied diet should not need to supplement with vitamins.

However, if you do not go out much, cover up when you do or have dark skin pigmentation, your levels of vitamin D – a vitamin synthesized under the skin on exposure to sunlight – could be low. Abdominal pain is a possible symptom of this deficiency. Exposing yourself to five or ten minutes of mild sunlight daily can help. Vitamin D is also found in margarine, butter, oily fish and liver. However, if your levels are low your doctor might advise taking high-dose vitamin D for a short while. Public Health England advises that a vitamin D supplement should be considered during winter months in the UK.

You probably can get all the vitamin C you need (around 40 mg) in half an orange, but supplements can contain high concentrations. Only 3,000 mg (3 g) of vitamin C a day can result in abdominal pain, nausea and diarrhoea – so take care.

Minerals

Magnesium supplements can cause diarrhoea, and both calcium supplements and iron tablets can cause constipation or diarrhoea, depending on the individual. Take them only if advised by a healthcare provider, and ask your pharmacist for a more 'gut-friendly' option if you experience such a reaction.

Note that high-dose magnesium supplements are sometimes sold as a 'bowel cleanse'. These are not recommended. A 'cleansed' bowel is *not* a healthy bowel. Good bacteria belong in it!

Nucleotides

These are components of DNA, the building blocks of our bodies' cells, and the idea behind nucleotide supplementation is to help counter the rapid turnover of cells in the digestive tract of people with IBS-D. However, the evidence for their effectiveness is currently weak; people without IBS also have a rapid turnover of large bowel cells – which is a normal occurrence – and some nucleotides contain FODMAPs in the form of inulin (fructans).

Prebiotics

These 'functional' foods are FODMAPs, so not all will tolerate them. That said, one prebiotic has been developed that can boost healthy bacterial populations without the side effects of gas and fermentation. It is called Bimuno® and contains a patented type of GOS that feeds friendly bacteria in the gut. More research is needed, but in a small study a 3.5 g daily dose was found to improve stool consistency, flatulence and bloating. It is available from high street pharmacies and online.

Digestive enzymes

There are a number of products on the market containing these. Those with diabetes should check with their doctor before trialling them, as they can alter blood sugar levels and some may affect other medications.

For fructose

Xylose isomerase is an enzyme that helps convert fructose to glucose for absorption. It is commercially available as Xylosolv® through a few online outlets. It has been found to be effective in doses of three capsules per 25 g fructose, though it should be pointed out that the research was funded by the company behind the enzyme. That said, you could try it if you are eating out and finding it more challenging to avoid high-fructose foods.

However, reducing fructose intake might be a more suitable option for people who need to manage their weight, as using a digestive enzyme may lead to an increase in calorie uptake.

For lactose

The digestive enzyme lactase helps with lactose digestion, and is widely available in supplemental form.

Reports of effectiveness vary, but it may be a suitable option when consumption of lactose is unavoidable, perhaps when travelling or in social situations. Versions with coated capsules, that can survive the stomach acid, are believed to be more effective than other options such as chewable tablets.

Lactase drops, widely available from health food stores or via the internet, can be added to ordinary milk to reduce lactose content, following 24 hours' refrigeration.

For GOS

A product called Beano® has been developed containing alpha galactosidase, an enzyme that helps digest this FODMAP. It is available from online pharmacies. It should not be taken by individuals with a rare condition called galactosaemia.

For gluten

There are a number on the market, such as Gluten-Zyme and GlutenEase, but there is little evidence to support their use in NCGS. They categorically do *not* help with coeliac disease, for which they are entirely useless.

Unvalidated diets for IBS

Any dietitian's aim is to ensure you obtain the nutrition you need while remaining symptom-free. Recommendations will be based on evidence – facts the medical profession has established through thorough research. Studies are always continuing in any medical field, which is why advice can change as we learn more. Good science and medicine moves with the research – it adapts to what we learn.

The idea of a 'quick fix' for any kind of difficulty is attractive. Celebrity endorsements and gushing media coverage make the latest fad diets appealing. But when public figures and 'wellness' bloggers advocate extreme or alternative diets to the masses without explaining the possible risks associated with them, the consumer is denied fully informed choice, and this is where danger lies. Testimonies sound powerful but are merely anecdotes, *not* medical research. They are vulnerable to the placebo effect – experiencing a positive outcome, due to the expectation of having one – but that may not last, long term. The reason fad diets come and go is because they don't work, but another one is always around the corner to take the place of the latest departed false promise!

The key point in IBS, as you have seen earlier in this chapter and in the last, is that dietary treatments have to be tailored to individuals, depending on their own responses to foods and their personal circumstances.

Below, we look at some of the diets you may have come across. All should be avoided, as they risk setting you back in your health, and may have other risks – such as malnutrition and a negative effect on your microbiome.

Raw food diet

This consists of a diet largely of food that has not been heated or cooked to greater than 40–50 °C; it is usually vegan and excludes beans and pulses. Its premise is that cooking destroys nutrients and enzymes, but this is flawed, as a varied diet of cooked and raw food gives you all the nutrition you need and some nutrients are more available to the body when cooked. Furthermore, the body is perfectly capable of producing its own enzymes. Advocates also believe it to be more 'alkaline' (less acidic) in nature and that this is better for the body – a theory that has been discredited.

Followers reduce the quantity of processed foods, including high-FODMAP wheat products, by following the raw food plan, so this may be why some derive temporary benefit from it.

Specific carbohydrate diet (SCD)

This is a sort of 'low-FODMAP' diet; however, it severely limits all FODMAPs except the M of monosaccharides, meaning that it permits fructose. There are other rules and excluded foods too. There have been no trials into the diet's effectiveness in IBS. Following it may be needlessly restrictive and risks failing to diagnose a fructose malabsorption problem.

GAPS diet

This is adapted from the SCD, but excludes fructose and nutritious foods such as oats and quinoa, and was originally developed to treat those with autism, learning disabilities and psychological disorders, for example. GAPS stands for gut and psychology syndrome, a condition invented by the diet's creator, Natasha Campbell-McBride, who has not published any scientific case reports on her regimen, and there have been no rigorous studies conducted into this either. The plan is further characterized by unscientific ideas such as detoxification and false food-sensitivity testing methods.

Candida diet

Candida is a yeast, naturally present in our bodies. Some alternative practitioners hold that a 'hidden' overgrowth of candida may underlie some complaints such as tiredness, digestive upsets and food cravings – and there is a little evidence to support this. The regimen excludes sugar, alcohol, fruits, pulses, mushrooms, yeast-containing foods and other foods, and is based on the notion of 'starving' the candida in the body.

Paleo diet

This is the 'caveman' diet – eating only foods available to early people, in the form in which they ate them. It is based around meat, fish, nuts, vegetables and fruit. The premise is flawed, as prehistoric people had a varied diet, including grains – which are excluded in modern paleo diets – and lived a short life, anyway. Benefits felt are likely to be due to lower FODMAP intake because of wheat exclusion. The diet is pointlessly restrictive, potentially too high in meat and saturated fat, and too low in complex carbohydrates.

Low-lectin diet

Wheat, peanut, beans, pulses and nightshade vegetables (such as potato, tomato and peppers) contain proteins called lectins, which some researchers believe can trigger bowel upsets. Many high-lectin foods are also high-FODMAP foods, making research difficult in this area, and the diet has not yet been tested for IBS so can't be recommended.

'Detox' and 'cleansing' diets

So-called detox regimens typically exclude wheat, dairy and sweet foods, which are high-FODMAP foods. Our liver and kidneys 'detoxify' any toxins in our body perfectly efficiently, and dietary restrictions offer no additional benefits to this function. Some plans include elements of fasting – but such short-term regimens are difficult to maintain, may make symptoms worse and will never offer a permanent solution.

Aloe vera is sometimes recommended by alternative therapists for its reputed cleansing benefits, but NICE guidelines say it should not be offered as a treatment in IBS. Its consumption can lead to electrolyte (salt) disturbances in the blood.

Therapists may also suggest juicing. Drinking fruit and vegetable juice – within the limits set by your reduced FODMAP diet, if you are on one – is fine. But substantially increasing your intake is more likely to worsen your IBS symptoms than benefit them. Consume whole vegetables or fruits instead.

6

Managing dietary changes

Following on from the support and advice you have received from your dietitian, you may have been subsequently advised to follow a restricted, altered or slightly modified diet – perhaps due to the identification of one or more food intolerances.

Your dietitian should have given you information on recipes, safe and nutritious foods and other lifestyle tips, but the reality of managing a new diet on your own may make you nervous.

Here we look at shopping for food and eating out – practical management of your food requirements, restrictions and diet, and its effects on your lifestyle.

Food labelling

Your dietitian may have impressed upon you the usefulness of home-cooked meals with safe ingredients in managing your symptoms, but while preparing your meals from scratch is terrific and should be done regularly, in the modern world, with busy lifestyles, this isn't always practical – and this means you will have to buy processed or prepacked foods. With any dietary restrictions, though, must come careful label-reading and scrutinizing.

Compulsory information

Some information must be given on labels. This includes a descriptive name of the product, a list of the ingredients (with any allergens emphasized, usually in bold), a 'best before' or 'use by' date, and the name and address of the manufacturer or importer of the product.

With only a few exceptions, nutritional information must be provided. The mandatory information, in order, is as follows, and applies to 100 g or 100 ml of product:

- Energy in kilojoules (kJ) or kilocalories (kcal) (popularly referred to as 'calories')
- Fat in grams
  - of which saturates
- Carbohydrate in grams
  - of which sugars
- Protein in grams
- Salt in grams.

Optional information

This includes serving suggestions and, in certain circumstances, country of origin.

Nutritional information may be supplemented with mono-unsaturated and polyunsaturated fats, cholesterol, polyols, starch, fibre, vitamins and minerals.

Food allergens

Although all ingredients must be provided on ingredients labels, the sources of some ingredients may not be clear or obvious – 'flavourings' or 'spices', for example. According to European legislation, however, certain foods must be named in the ingredients list – and not only when they are present as whole foods but also when they are the source of an ingredient.

There are 14 such foods or food groups and they are often described as the main food allergens, chosen because they are the most commonly and dangerously problematic ones for people who react to foods.

The full list of allergens is:

- celery (and celeriac)
- cereals containing gluten – barley, oats, rye and wheat
- crustaceans (such as crab, lobster, prawns)
- eggs
- fish
- lupin
- milk (including lactose)
- molluscs (such as mussels, squid)
- mustard

- nuts (almonds, cashew, walnuts, for example)
- peanuts
- sesame seeds
- soya beans
- sulphur dioxide and sulphites.

The 14 allergens should be highlighted in ingredients lists when they are present, in order to make them stand out more clearly. Most manufacturers use **bold** to highlight them, but some use underlining, *italics*, CAPITALS, a different colour or a combination of these.

There are some exemptions to this rule, such as glucose syrups derived from wheat, or maltodextrin, as they are considered no risk to those with allergies or coeliac disease because processing has removed the problematic proteins.

Although it is not a requirement, many manufacturers include an additional allergy advice statement. Such statements direct consumers towards the list of ingredients and explain the method used for highlighting allergens. For example, 'Allergy advice: for allergens, including cereals containing gluten, see ingredients in **bold**.'

Non-prepacked food

Businesses selling non-prepacked food sold loose at bakeries, takeaways, butchers and deli counters, for example, also have to provide information on which of the 14 allergens they contain.

This can be provided via a chalkboard or information pack, for example. It can also be supplied orally via a member of staff, though if this is the case it must be signposted that customers should ask for it, and the information should be consistent and verifiable, if challenged.

Food businesses are not permitted to plead ignorance about the allergens their foods contain, and neither can they declare that all their products 'may contain' the key allergens. They are legally obliged to provide accurate information.

A gluten-free claim can be made for loose foods, but the same standards as for prepacked foods apply.

Note that there is no obligation to provide a full list of ingredients for non-prepacked foods – though many will.

Precautionary 'may contain' labelling

This labelling is also voluntary and unregulated. Examples of so-called advisory labelling include 'may contain traces of gluten' or 'made in a factory that handles nuts'.

Such labelling may be used by manufacturers for two reasons: to warn the public that certain allergens, although not intentionally added as ingredients, might have accidentally contaminated a product or one or more of its ingredients somewhere along the harvesting, transporting or manufacturing line; and also to disclaim any liability should a customer suffer a reaction.

Manufacturers are advised that such labelling should be used only when, following a thorough risk assessment, they believe there is a real risk of cross-contamination. Some are overcautious, which frustrates many who react to foods. They are generally more relevant to those with food allergies and coeliac disease than to those with a FODMAP intolerance.

'Free from' foods

These are processed products free from one or more of the ingredients that would normally be present in the food's non-'free from' equivalent.

These ingredients are typically the food allergens, but increasingly 'sugar-free' and 'additive-free' foods are being marketed.

There's been a huge growth in 'free from' foods in recent years, partly fuelled by the increase in diagnoses of various food allergies and intolerances and an interest in vegetarian or vegan diets, but also by many choosing to eliminate certain foods from their diets for perceived health reasons.

You'll find many wheat-free and/or dairy-free products in the 'free from' aisle of the supermarket – a section reserved for specialist foods for allergies and intolerances and vegan foods. Try speciality ethnic stores for foods such as buckwheat and rice noodles. Health food shops are good, as are online stores such as Ocado, Goodness Direct and Amazon. The best online stores allow you to filter out by allergen, so you can choose 'milk-free', 'sugar-free' and 'wheat-free' for instance (see the Useful addresses section).

There are downsides to 'free from' foods, though. First, they can be dearer, because of the cost of allergen testing and specialist ingredients and the difficulty of manufacture, among other reasons. Second, they're not always the healthiest of products. Some can be higher in fat and sugar, and may require a host of additives. They're terrific in helping you make the transition to your new diet or for occasional treats, but don't rely on them too much.

Besides, many 'ordinary' foods, not specifically designed for those on restricted diets, will be suitable.

Food directories

King's College London's booklet on suitable products for the low-FODMAP diet is only available to registered dietitians, but if your dietitian is using the KCL plan, it should be available to you to consult.

Coeliac UK's annual *Food and Drink Directory* lists around 10,000 gluten-free products – although not all will be low FODMAP. Updated every January, it is divided into sections such as 'free from' products, everyday products and supermarket own-brand products.

The Coeliac Society of Ireland produces the *Food List*, the Irish equivalent of the *Food and Drink Directory*.

Shopping for a low-FODMAP diet

When it comes to wholefoods, you'll have been told by your dietitian which are suitable and safe and which you may need to moderate or avoid, but what about processed foods?

Although awareness of the plan is growing, few food manufacturers are stating if their products are high, medium or low in FODMAPs. There is a new 'FODMAP Friendly' certification programme (see <www.FODMAP.com>), with a green logo (see Figure 6.1), and another 'Low FODMAP Certified' logo from Monash University, which is blue. Both may come into common use soon.

It may not be easy to deduce the FODMAP suitability of a processed food. Look for any ingredients listed as high-FODMAP foods in Table 4.1 on pages 44–5 and 'FODMAP types' on pages 45–7.

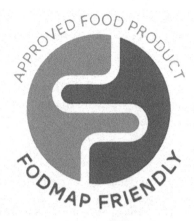

Figure 6.1 'FODMAP Friendly' certification logo

The higher an ingredient is listed, the more of it is present. If you're avoiding wheat and it is the first ingredient of, for example, a baked product, it will probably be a high-FODMAP food. If a high-FODMAP ingredient comes lower down in the list, though, it may be safe.

Onion and garlic

Look out especially for these – you'll typically find them in stock cubes, soups, dressings, gravy and ready meals. Because they are not 'top 14' allergens, terms such as 'flavouring' or 'seasoning' could potentially include derivatives of onion or garlic, although these are likely to be in low levels. Bear in mind, though, that during the elimination phase of the diet, onion and garlic should be avoided in all amounts, so check with manufacturers if necessary.

Milk and lactose

Milk is one of the 14 key allergens so must be highlighted on labelling. The ingredient milk itself will be highlighted, but if the ingredient is cream, yogurt or butter, either the ingredient may be highlighted, or the word 'milk' may appear alongside, highlighted.
So, for example, 'cream (**milk**)' and '**cream**' are both possible.
Other milk ingredients must feature the word 'milk'. For example, 'whey (**milk**)'.

If you can't confirm that a milk ingredient is low FODMAP, it is safer to avoid, especially if high in the list of ingredients.

Sugar

Sucrose or table sugar is safe but if the type of 'sugar' is not explained on a label, check with the manufacturer. Watch out for the sugars and syrups listed on page 45.

Breads

One hundred per cent sourdough spelt bread is low FODMAP – but not gluten-free. Naturally occurring yeasts and bacteria are used in the dough, and the traditional slow production method ensures FODMAPs are drastically reduced. The resulting texture is more like that of wheaten bread, but with a sour note. Search artisanal producers at the Real Bread Campaign's site (<www.sustainweb.org/realbread>). Note their sourdough classifications: only type I or II (not III) is suitable – avoid spelt and rye blends.

Gluten-free breads tend to be low FODMAP, but check ingredients and be wary of 'flavoured' varieties, such as garlic bread. These breads can be an acquired taste, though. There are many varieties – such as ciabattas, pittas, rolls and wraps, in seeded, white and brown. 'Refreshing' or toasting breads improves flavour.

One hundred per cent teff or millet flour breads are not suitable, though these ingredients in combination with others will be. Other ingredients you may see are:

- **partially invert sugar syrup,** which can contain varying amounts of fructose but is unlikely to be found in large quantity in gluten-free bread;
- **pea protein,** which has been recently tested as low FODMAP so should be safe;
- **concentrated fruit juice,** which can contain apple;
- **Codex wheat starch,** which is 'deglutenized' wheat starch, with under 20 parts per million gluten. It is mostly used in prescription breads for coeliacs, but may turn up in on-shelf products. Not yet tested.

NB: small amounts of FODMAPs in gluten-free breads should be fine for most. Try two slices at first, or even just one of any bread containing Codex. If you react to one brand, try another.

Polyol ingredients

The sweeteners sorbitol, maltitol, xylitol, isomalt and mannitol crop up in sugar-free products, chewing gum and confectionery, so-called diabetic foods, sweet processed foods, frozen desserts and sweetened medicines such as cough syrups or throat lozenges.

Fructans ingredients

Watch out for terms such as fructo-oligosaccharide (FOS) or oligo-fructose. Prebiotic ingredients such as inulin (derived from chicory) should also be avoided.

For advice on wheat avoidance, see 'Shopping for a gluten-free diet', below.

Shopping for a gluten-free diet

To some extent, how careful you need to be with shopping is dependent on how sensitive you are to gluten. If you have coeliac disease or wheat allergy, then you have to be absolutely strict; if you have NCGS, we don't know how careful you need to be so it might be prudent to avoid gluten altogether.

Wheat, barley, rye and oat labelling

These grains are defined as 'gluten-containing cereals' under labelling law, and have to be highlighted in ingredients.

- If the grain features in the ingredient's name, only the grain should be highlighted – '**wheat** flour', for example.
- If the ingredient's name partly consists of the grain, either the whole word should be highlighted or just the grain – '**oatmeal** flour' or '**oat**meal flour', for instance.
- Where the grain does not feature in the ingredient's name, it should be highlighted alongside, as in 'couscous (**wheat**)'.
- The word 'gluten' is usually optional, but if used it will *not* be highlighted, so either '**rye** flour (gluten)' or '**rye** flour' may be used, for example.

If there are no gluten-containing cereals listed in the ingredients and no precautionary labelling mentioning a gluten grain (see page 74), then the product should be gluten-free (GF).

'Gluten-free' labelling

Unlike any other 'free from' claim, gluten-free is defined in law. It means less than 20 parts per million – or 0.002 per cent – of gluten, which is extremely low and research suggests those with coeliac disease can tolerate.

Manufacturers carrying the 'gluten-free' message are claiming that their products contain 0.002 per cent gluten or under. Another badge of safety is the Coeliac UK Crossed Grain certification symbol (see Figure 6.2). The absence of a 'gluten-free' claim or symbol does not necessarily mean a product is not GF, however.

Precautionary 'may contain' labelling

Other than 'may contain wheat / gluten' you may also see expressions such as 'may not be suitable for coeliacs' to indicate possible contamination.

Coeliac UK say they can contact manufacturers to talk through the actual risk, and the charity does sometimes list such products in its annual handbook, the *Food and Drink Directory* (see page 70), following discussions with them about production facilities and measures to minimize cross-contamination. If you're concerned, contact the charity or the manufacturer for further information. It may be that a product is safe.

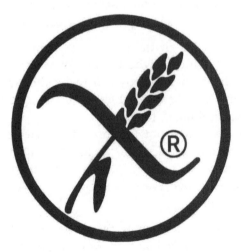

Figure 6.2 The Coeliac UK Crossed Grain certification logo

'Wheat-free'

A product bearing this claim might *not* be gluten-free, since it could contain rye or barley.

Note that a 'wheat-free' claim is occasionally used wrongly on products containing spelt, which is a form of wheat.

Oats

For the purposes of allergy labelling legislation, oats are considered gluten-containing cereals – and you will therefore see the word 'oat' highlighted in ingredients. Evidence suggests, however, that the 'gluten' protein in oats (called avenin) is safe at modest levels for most with gluten sensitivities.

That said, most commercial oats are contaminated with wheat flour and may therefore trigger symptoms in people with coeliac disease (it's uncertain in the case of NCGS). Special 'gluten-free' oats – grown and processed well away from potential wheat contamination – are now widely available. They are low FODMAP.

Shopping for other diets

For various reasons – such as food allergies, or for cultural or ethical reasons – you may avoid other foods or follow a particular diet, and this can complicate the identification of safe foods for you – especially when you have to follow a low-FODMAP and/or gluten-free diet in tandem.

One way to find products online is to use search functions and filters, such as 'gluten-free' and 'kosher' on Ocado's website.

Dairy-free and milk-free

As a key allergen, 'milk' (or 'yogurt', 'cream' or 'butter') has to be emphasized on labels (see pages 71–2).

There are many plant-based milk alternatives, but not all are suitable for all diets. Check ingredients for high-FODMAP apple juice, and choose a calcium-fortified option. Table 6.1 shows a selection.

Vegan cheese alternatives are not always low-FODMAP options. Check for onion and garlic flavourings and all sources of added vegetable fibres.

Table 6.1 Some alternatives to milk

Vegan milk replacement	Low-FODMAP 'milk'	Gluten-free?	Fortified with calcium?
Alpro Almond Unsweetened Fresh	Yes	Yes	Yes
Alpro Hazelnut Original	Yes	Yes	Yes
Alpro Coconut Original	Yes	Yes	Yes
KoKo Dairy Free Original	(125 ml or a small glass)	Yes	Yes
Good Hemp Unsweetened	Yes	Yes	Yes
Ecomil Hemp Drink	Yes	Yes	No
Alpro Soya Original Fresh	(60 ml)	Yes	Yes
Provamel Soya Natural	(60 ml)	Yes	No*
Oatly Oat Drink	Yes	No	No
Oatly Oat Drink with calcium	Yes	No	Yes
Rude Health Oat Milk	Yes	Yes	No
Provitamil Oat Milk	Yes	No	Yes

* Calcium-added versions contain apple concentrate, so are not low-FODMAP options.

Unless you have a milk allergy or a strict moral objection, you won't need to worry about 'may contain traces of milk' warnings, which are common on products such as dark chocolate, often made without milk.

Jewish kosher

Following religious restrictions and specific diets for food intolerances can be challenging. Kosher rules are complex and are not just a matter of eating foods approved via the Beth Din. The status of products can change depending on manufacturers' use of ingredients, so check regularly.

Email and text alerts and telephone information are available from the Kashrut London Beth Din. Their site states the pareve status of foods: <www.kosher.org.uk/koshersearch>.

The Manchester Beth Din site is also useful: <www.mbd.org.uk/site/kosher-products>.

Suitable low-FODMAP products or brands that are kosher-certified include:

- Barkat gluten- and wheat-free matzo crackers; some supermarkets stock a brand called Yehuda, imported from Israel, and made with potato and tapioca;
- Yarden Aubergine and Mayonnaise;
- Mr Freed's Tuna Salad and Mr Freed's Coleslaw, both gluten-free and dairy-free;
- Eskal brand, which is kosher-certified and includes gluten-free pretzels and other baked goods;
- gluten- and wheat-free bagels – such as by Genius, BFree and Goodness Grains – which are increasingly available, but check on pareve status;
- Rizopia organic brown rice pasta;
- BFree gluten-free breads, wraps and rolls;
- Bute Island (Sheese – dairy-free);
- Schwartz Cheddar, Sol Edam slices, The Milk Company Original Mozzarella Rolled (these are Chalav Yisrael supervised milk products);
- Doves Farm flours, pasta and biscuits (chocolate, lemon and ginger);
- Kellogg's Cornflakes and Rice Krispies (neither is gluten-free) and Kallo Puffed Rice.

Some high-FODMAP products:

- Cohens Bakery Buckingham Boulangerie Challa
- Rakusen's baked beans and cracker ranges and matza meal
- Scrumshus Granola, Kellogg's Bran Flakes
- Mr Freed's Fish Balls
- Camp Chicory and Coffee Essence.

These lists are not exhaustive and the KLBD's *Really Jewish Food Guide* has a good selection of 'free from' products suitable for the low-FODMAP diet.

NB: Supervised kosher milk is not likely to be lactose-free. Lactose drops are a possibility, but note that the drops are not explicitly approved. Speak with your local Beth Din or rabbi for advice.

South Asian

Low-FODMAP foods:

- aloo or bateta (potato)
- bringles, baingan or brinjal (aubergine)
- chakri, chakli or murruku (fried dough snacks; make with rice flour but no ajwain – which is untested – or garlic)
- coriander
- hing, anjanda or asafoetida (NB: not always wheat-free)
- huldi (turmeric)
- keema (minced meat curry – make it without onion and garlic)
- kesar (saffron)
- kheera, taar or kakadi (cucumber)
- machchi or machali (fish)
- methi (fenugreek)
- murgi (chicken)
- Natco corn meal fine
- palak or sag (spinach).

High-FODMAP foods:

- aloo gobi (potato and cauliflower curry) (make without onion, garlic and cauliflower)
- amchur (mango powder)*
- ata or atta (bread)
- bhaturas (leavened bread)
- bhindi (okra or ladies' fingers) (limit to six pods)
- channa or channa dhal (chickpea)**
- chappati, rothi, chupatti
- dhal (pulse-based curry)
- dhiwada or dahi bhalle (urid dhal) (pulses)
- ganthia (chickpea flour snack)
- gram or besan (chickpea flour)**
- jalebi (wheat-based sweet snack)
- kheer (rice pudding)
- masoor (red lentils)
- mathi or menda puri
- mung dhal (pulse)
- naan (bread)

- paneer (Indian cheese)*
- poori or puries (unleavened bread)
- rajma or lobia (kidney beans)
- rawaa (black-eyed beans)**
- tuver dhal (dried split pigeon peas)
- tuver green (pigeon peas)
- urid dhal (black lentils).**

* Untested, but probably a high-FODMAP food.
** Two rinsed tablespoons are permitted.

You can, of course, use lactose-free milk and gluten-free flours to make many of the wheat-flour and milk-based foods above.

African–Caribbean

Some foods have not been tested for FODMAPs, but others are suitable, so some traditional meals can be consumed.

Low-FODMAP foods:

- ackee (tinned)
- breadfruit
- callaloo (tinned)
- cassava (limit to 100 g)
- cinnamon
- coconut milk (limit to 100 ml)
- dumplings (made from yam only)
- jeera or zera (cumin)
- plantain
- sweet potato (limit to 70 g)
- yam.

High-FODMAP foods:

- black-eyed peas*
- coconut water
- Jamaican crackers (try GF crackers instead)
- jerk seasoning
- peas (kidney beans)*
- pigeon peas.*

* Tinned rinsed beans are suitable – two tablespoons per portion.

Managing on a budget

'Free from' foods and some low-FODMAP wholefoods are expensive, so how can we make a restricted diet more affordable? Here are 20 ideas.

1 Buy in bulk anything that doesn't perish quickly, particularly basics such as rice, polenta and buckwheat, in ethnic supermarkets especially, where you may also get very good deals on spices, wheat-free flours and noodles.
2 Make the most of special offers or promotional weeks at supermarkets – including discount supermarkets – for particular low-FODMAP or wheat-free foods.
3 Misshapen and in-season fruit and vegetables may be cheaper – and tastier!
4 Check the 'yellow sticker' mark-down offers – much food about to fall out of date can be frozen, including 'free from' breads.
5 Base meals on affordable carbohydrates, such as potatoes and rice.
6 Make your own sweet treats – using safe foods such as dark chocolate, peppermint, cinnamon and 100 per cent maple syrup.
7 Make your own wheat-free flour blends by mixing wheat-free flours, bought in bulk.
8 Don't be shy of using coupons and joining supermarkets' points schemes.
9 Although typically restricted to coeliacs only, some gluten-free brands may be willing to send taster samples of products if you are on a low-FODMAP diet.
10 Plan your food for the week and shop accordingly. Don't shop on an empty stomach – you'll be more likely to purchase unplanned items if you're hungry.
11 A cheaper cut of meat and low-FODMAP vegetables make a terrific casserole.
12 Buy oats (gluten-free if necessary) in bulk, and make your own muesli using modest amounts of low-FODMAP dried fruit and nuts and seeds.
13 Frozen and tinned fruit and vegetables can be cheaper – but the preserving juice in tinned fruit may be a high-FODMAP one.

14 Avoid 'free from' sauces – they typically contain onion and garlic and are not a great deal different from ordinary sauces. Instead, make your own and thicken with cornflour.

15 Shop around and browse. Don't restrict yourself to 'free from' shelves. Visit aisles you wouldn't normally visit, where undiscovered bargains may lurk!

16 Online delivery can save time but check delivery costs before you buy. Some supermarkets offer cheaper delivery during usual office hours.

17 When cooking, bulk cook and freeze portions – which also saves on fuel costs.

18 Don't waste meat or vegetable scraps – instead, make your own stock, with a bay leaf and carrot. Skim off the fat when cooled, and freeze in small amounts.

19 Visit a market later in the day as stallholders often discount produce at around 5 p.m.

20 Visit farm shops – they can sell staples such as potatoes and eggs more cheaply.

Cooking low-FODMAP meals

Many of the recipes in your culinary repertoire will be adaptable to low-FODMAP (or other) diets. The 'free from' foods available – the wide array of wheat-free pastas or lactose-free, dairy-free products, for example – mean that staple meals need not be altered too much.

Try to use restrictions to get creative and introduce permitted foods and new dishes into your diet. There are recipes in Appendix 2.

Some foods, though, are harder to compensate for. Here are some ideas.

Onion

You can replace onion with chives or the green part of spring onions or leeks, although these do impart a slightly different flavour.

Another option for curries or sauces is to put a small pinch of an Indian spice called asafoetida (hing) into the hot oil for frying. It has a pungent smell but this disappears to leave a savoury oniony taste. Some asafoetida contains wheat flour, so check labels if you are coeliac or wheat allergic (those on a low-FODMAP diet should tolerate the tiny amounts used).

Garlic

Garlic is a high-FODMAP food, but garlic-infused oil is fine – provided it is clear, not cloudy – as garlic's FODMAP content is only soluble in water, not oil. Use it as a starting oil in frying. If you make your own, filter or remove fried pieces of garlic before adding other ingredients.

Mirepoix and soffritto

These are lightly fried mixed or chopped vegetables that are the base for many French and Italian dishes. They contain celery and carrot, but also onion and sometimes garlic. For a low-FODMAP alternative, omit the garlic and onion, and consider some fennel (under 50 g) or fennel seeds instead, for an unusual aniseed taste. You can also replace celery with chopped celeriac to further reduce FODMAP content. Strong dried herbs, such as rosemary, marjoram and thyme, can add another taste dimension.

Stock

Most stocks contain onion and garlic. If you have completed the reintroduction phase you might find you tolerate the small amounts of FODMAPs in stock. If not, you could use cooking water from low-FODMAP vegetables and/or boil chicken or beef bones to make your own and freeze it. You could also add some wine to food where you would normally use liquid stocks.

Eating out

Having a dietary restriction shouldn't stop you eating out, but it can make it more challenging.

Improved allergen regulations have meant awareness has improved, especially of wheat- and gluten-free diets. All caterers and food service providers are obliged to tell you – either on menus or otherwise on request – about the presence of any of the 14 allergens (see page 67) in their food, but do not have to declare other ingredients – although in practice they should be able to. This does *not* mean an outlet is obliged to serve you a 'free from' meal. That said, many can and do.

Although it's not always possible, preplanning will help.

- **Go online** Most outlets have websites on which menus can be viewed or downloaded.
- **Phone ahead** Speak with the head waiter, chef or a senior member of the waiting staff.
- **Give examples** If you have complicated dietary requirements, explain which kinds of meals might suit you, how other meals can be adapted or how specific simple dishes can be prepared – for instance, asking for meat to be grilled, not fried, if fatty foods upset your digestion. You don't have to explain your symptoms or condition: you just have to talk about food and convey that it is a need.
- **Book a table** Ask for one with easy access to a toilet, if this makes you more comfortable.
- **Get fellow diners on side** Let the friends and family you're dining with know about your circumstances, so they can support you as needed.

And what about when you arrive?

- If you called ahead, ask to meet the person you spoke with. Go through your conversation again, confirming what you agreed.
- If you haven't prebooked or vetted the eatery, inform a member of staff immediately about your requirements. Check if suitable options are available.
- Read menus carefully. Never let hunger or impatience get the better of judgement. Ask staff to clarify ambiguities and specify safe meals – possibly recommended by the chefs.
- Don't become complacent. Go through the usual checks in restaurants at which you've previously dined and you have come to 'know'.
- Be polite throughout. Make a point at the end of the meal of thanking staff for catering for you.

Low-FODMAP diet

Chefs and restaurant staff may not yet be aware of this relatively new diet!

You may have to scrutinize available ingredients carefully and question staff closely. Grilled plain fish or meat are good options, with plain rice and freshly cooked potato, which are ideal starchy components. Egg dishes, such as omelettes, can be fine if onion- and garlic-free. Ask about any sauces, stocks and dressings. Gluten-free meals (see below) might be suitable.

Sushi is a probable good option, and accompanying wasabi and ginger are suitable flavourings, but check for vegetarian rolls made with high-FODMAP ingredients such as garlic and onion.

Gluten-free

Many outlets now have gluten-free menus or use 'GF' to highlight menu options.

Coeliac UK offer accreditation to organizations catering to gluten-free diners. Their GF symbol (see Figure 6.3) tells you that the food service provider adheres to the charity's gluten-free standard, which covers all aspects of food preparation as well as guaranteeing that training has taken place.

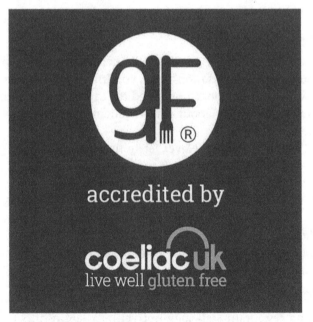

Figure 6.3 The Coeliac UK GF Catering Accreditation logo

Other diets

Diets such as vegetarian, vegan, kosher or halal can pose greater difficulties, although there are a number of restaurants catering to these particular cuisines.

Good vegan options might include risotto and low-FODMAP vegetables, or rice-stuffed pepper, unless containing onion or garlic.

Drinking and alcohol

Alcohol can stimulate contractions of the digestive system. A high intake can irritate the tissues of the digestive tract and can cause serious complications with the liver and pancreas. It can also result in stomach ache, diarrhoea, sickness and vomiting. Symptoms of diarrhoea and IBS are associated with binge drinking (defined as double the recommended guidelines in one episode).

Government guidelines issued in 2016 advise both men and women to drink no more than 14 units evenly spread through a week – equivalent to six pints of beer, seven glasses of wine or 14 glasses of 40 per cent spirits (a glass is 25 ml) – and at least two alcohol-free days a week are recommended. Heavy drinking should be avoided. There is no healthy level of intake. Pregnant women should not drink at all. See Drink Aware (<www.drinkaware.co.uk>) for further information.

In people with IBS lower intakes than these are advisable, especially of gassy or carbonated drinks or mixers.

Reducing intake

You could have a glass of wine, for example, with your main meal, or ask for a spritzer to make a longer drink. Order a spritzer with your starter and allow it to go a little flat before drinking it if you suffer from bloating. Using an implement such as a straw or cocktail stirrer to mix your drink will help to disperse the gas it contains, but don't drink through the straw.

FODMAPs and gluten in drinks

Most alcohol is low FODMAP except rum, sweet wine, sherry and port, which could contain fructose.

Mixers with artificial sweeteners are likely to be better than those sweetened with glucose–fructose syrups.

Watch the amount of fruit cocktails you have, if you have fructose intolerance – one small glass (100 ml) of pure fruit juice containing low-FODMAP fruits is usually the maximum portion advised.

Some people struggle with lager, possibly because of the gas it contains. Gluten-free beer is available.

Bar snacks

Some low-FODMAP options include:

- olives (check dressing has no garlic and onion);
- peanuts;
- plain or salt and vinegar crisps;
- Peppadew (choose mild if chilli gives you symptoms);
- gluten-free pretzels and breadsticks.

At work

If you have a staff canteen, the same advice applies as when eating out – as do the same regulations – but the canteen may not be as well equipped to cater, especially in smaller companies. Some suggestions:

- jacket potato and tuna mayonnaise and green salad
- omelette (no onion) and green salad
- grilled chicken, meat, fish (no sauce)
- steak and jacket potato.

Bringing your own home-made lunch can be more cost-effective:

- gluten-free sandwiches with ham and white cabbage and carrot coleslaw
- rice or gluten-free pasta salad
- potato salad
- gluten-free wraps or pitta breads with salad and chicken, hard cheese or fish.

'On the go'

It can be tough when out and about to find suitable foods, and it is better to be prepared for this eventuality so that you are not tempted to eat unsuitable foods. Here are some ideas:

- fruit – banana, orange, small handful of grapes
- gluten-free breadsticks or crackers
- small handful of suitable nuts and seeds
- an occasional treat – crisps, flapjack (check ingredients), dark chocolate-coated rice cakes, rice bars, cornflake cakes.

Lactofree produce handy 20-ml long-life portions of milk, available from most larger supermarkets.

7

Emotional well-being

For many with IBS who have linked diet to their symptoms for some time, it has come as a comfort that their food intolerances have now been validated by the medical community. However, we know that IBS is not just a matter of changing what you eat.

In subsequent chapters we will look at physical well-being and offer practical advice to staying well. But in this chapter, we focus on psychological health and help you navigate everyday emotional challenges you may encounter.

Breathing

What could be more fundamental to life – and health – than breathing? Although it's a physical process, because the respiratory and cardiovascular systems are often directly affected by emotions it's appropriate to consider it here.

The most important muscle used in breathing is the diaphragm – a strong flat muscle attached to the lower edges of the ribs. It separates the chest and lungs from your stomach and bowel, and is shaped like the dome of an umbrella when relaxed.

Good breathing means moving air in and out of the chest and lungs with the minimum of effort and using the right muscles, ensuring your body receives the appropriate amount of oxygen.

As you inhale, the diaphragm contracts and moves downwards, drawing air into your lungs and causing your belly to expand and rise. As you exhale, it moves upwards, pushing air from your lungs.

It is the most instinctive form of breathing, practised naturally by mammals when they are relaxed. Our modern busy lives mean we often breathe from the chest – a state that is often associated with increased anxiety – rather than from the belly. It is only during increased activity that the upper chest should open up to draw in extra air.

Unless you are exercising, it's important you breathe in and out through your nose to help filter, warm and moisten the air. At rest you should be taking 8–12 breaths a minute.

Practising good breathing

This exercise is adapted with kind permission from Physiotherapy for Hyperventilation (<www.physiohypervent.org>).

1 Lie comfortably on your back with a pillow under your head and knees.
2 Place one hand on your stomach, the other relaxed by your side.
3 Gently close your mouth and keep your jaw loose.
4 Breathe in gently through your nose, feeling your tummy rise and expand. The breath should be unforced and silent. Your upper chest should be relaxed and not moving; place your hand on it to check from time to time.
5 Breathe out lightly through your nose if possible, without pushing, keeping your stomach relaxed.
6 Relax and pause at the end of each breath out.

As you repeat this sequence, be aware of any areas of tension in your body and concentrate on 'letting go', particularly jaw, neck, shoulders and hands.

Practise as often as you can. Try to do it a little and often – perhaps for three minutes every hour. Check the number of breaths you take per minute – each in–out cycle should last for six to eight seconds. As you practise, you will find your natural rhythm.

Progress to practising while sitting, then standing and finally walking. As your body adapts to this way of breathing, you will find it demands less time and energy and is more relaxing. Remember, the more practice, the sooner you will feel back in control of any stress.

Mouth breathing

Breathing through your mouth can increase the amount of air in your stomach, which can leave you feeling bloated and full. If you have difficulty when you try to breathe through your nose instead, see your doctor.

A gentle word on anxiety

Anxiety in the newly diagnosed is a problem for some, but not all, and this is a controversial topic among people with IBS. It's important that anxiety is recognized when present, so you can try treatments. It is best diagnosed by your GP.

Anxiety is the body's normal response to danger that prepares it for 'fight or flight'. It becomes a problem when it is out of proportion to the 'threat', or else experienced when no danger is present. Symptoms include racing heartbeat, shortness of breath, chest tightness, dry mouth, butterflies in the stomach, nausea, the urge to pass urine or empty the bowel, tremor, sweating and pins and needles.

Relaxation

'Relax!'

It's a command we've all heard many times, often from the mouths of family members or friends who seem far calmer than us. How is it that some people seem to be able to be relaxed for most of their lives, while others are jittery or anxious or restless at even the slightest provocation?

People often report that symptoms worsen when they feel stressed. It is common for people to experience diarrhoea when nervous – for an exam or interview, for instance. We also know that in around a third of those with IBS, stress is a major causative factor.

If this sounds like you, be consoled that all of us experience stress from time to time. It is completely natural. But if you have IBS it can trigger symptoms, or the worsening of existing ones. Obeying the command to 'relax' may be an obvious solution, but there is more to relaxation than merely willing yourself to do so. You have to work at it and, like good breathing, practise it. Putting pressure on yourself to relax can merely increase the stress – so don't worry if you find you're not very good at it at first! You will get better.

Incorporating simple techniques for relaxation into your daily life – much as you might make time for lunch or to enjoy the evening's TV – can work wonders. Try some of the following, and record yourself reading out the instructions and play them back so you can concentrate better on the routines.

Two-minute calm down

Perform this in a quiet place.

1 Have a full-body stretch, then sit on a comfortable chair.
2 Position yourself so your feet are firmly planted on the floor, with hips loose and hands cupped on your lap or palms flat on the knees.
3 Slide your bottom to the back of the chair. Keep shoulders loose.
4 Perform a chin tuck – bringing your chin to your chest – for five seconds, and return.
5 Drop your jaw for three seconds, and return.
6 Stretch out your fingers – one hand at a time.
7 Practise good breathing, feeling your waist expand gently and noticing the relaxed pause at the end of each out breath.
8 To still your busy brain, concentrate on mentally placing numbers on the relaxed pause phases. Don't try to stop your thoughts – simply let the numerals take centre-stage.
9 Count each full breathing cycle from one to ten, then back to one, breathing low and slow – that is, breathe in, breathe out, count one; then breathe in, breathe out, count two, and so on.
10 Stretch, smile and go back to what you were doing.

Action and distraction relaxation

This is useful for when one symptom dominates and threatens to ruin your day.

1 Sit, stand or lie down – as you wish.
2 Keep lips together, jaw relaxed, legs loose, neck central and relaxed.
3 Practise good breathing, with eyes closed or focused mid-distance.
4 In your mind, ask yourself questions about your awareness of parts of your body and clothing, and focus for at least 20 seconds on each. For example: 'Can I feel the watch on my wrist?' 'Can I feel the collar on my neck?' 'Can I feel the ring

on my finger?' – then continue with 'Can I feel the earring in my right ear?' 'Can I feel the sock on my left foot?' and so on.

5 Finish with a gentle body stretch when the dominating symptom subsides.

Repeat any time one symptom gets 'too loud' . . .

Visualization techniques

Combining belly breathing – when you have become more adept at it – with some visualization can further boost relaxation. Again, this can be performed seated or lying, but close your eyes.

1 Establish a rhythm of belly breathing.
2 Visualize any relaxing scene – a gentle waterfall, perhaps, or a field of poppies, whatever soothes you.
3 After a while, embroider the fantasy with detail – hear the buzz of grasshoppers or imagine the warmth of the sun, for example.
4 Ensure your breathing stays in good rhythm.
5 'Leave' your scene slowly when you feel relaxed and ready.

Again, this takes practice, and you may take a while to find your right 'place'.

Progressive muscular relaxation

This is a sequence of targeted exercises whereby you individually tense and release groups of muscles in your body – but never to the point of pain. Relax the tension if it does hurt or skip any parts of your body that are tender or injured. If you have muscular difficulties or conditions, consult your doctor first.

1 Lie or sit comfortably, with eyes closed.
2 Establish a rhythm of diaphragmatic breathing.
3 Begin with the muscles in your forehead. Either force brows to furrow or 'frown' or else raise eyebrows high. Hold to a slow count of five (a full cycle of either inhalation or exhalation). Then release and make an effort to note and enjoy the feeling of relaxation as tension subsides.
4 After five or ten seconds, screw up your eyes tight. (Use only your eye muscles, not those in your cheek or around your mouth.) Hold for five, then relax, as before.

5 After five or ten seconds, flare your nostrils and/or wrinkle your nose. Hold for five, then relax.
6 Progress in this vein. Smile widely, lifting your cheeks, repeating the procedure.
7 Tense your jaw.
8 Move to your neck, taking particular care with this part of the body: stretch it gently left, then release, then right, and release, and back, and release, and forward, and release.
9 Shrug your shoulders up to your ears, and hold.
10 Clench your fists.
11 Flex your biceps.
12 Push your shoulders back (as if to make your shoulder blades touch).
13 Flex your pectoral muscles.
14 Tighten your stomach muscles, pulling in.
15 Tighten your buttocks.
16 Press your knees together to tighten thighs.
17 Tighten calves.
18 Point toes towards you.
19 Point toes away from you.

That's it! Enjoy the feeling for as long as you like, and perhaps return to any parts of the body you feel are still tense as they may need more work.

Also, you can make the exercise more specific, focusing on any particular stubborn knots and tailor the routine to your needs. For instance, if you type a lot, you may like to work on your fingers individually.

This exercise takes more time, so set aside half an hour.

Massage

This can be very relaxing – if you see a professional masseur or masseuse, do let him or her know of your condition beforehand, and seek advice from your healthcare advisor. Massage from a caring partner may be all you need, though.

You can also self-massage. It's best done after a warm bath and using some very gentle body oils, but can be very effective for stiffness of the neck, for example.

People power

Self-help is terrific, but sometimes you need other people in your life to support you and the benefits of interacting with family, friends and acquaintances should not be underestimated. It can make a real difference.

It is important friends and family recognize what a debilitating condition IBS can be and how they can help. Most people are more than willing to help but sometimes don't understand or appreciate what you would find helpful. Talk to them! And listen, too: a friend telling you that you cope with your situation well and empathizing with your situation can strengthen you.

Others' attitudes

It can be easy for family, friends and colleagues who live, work or socialize with a person who has IBS to dismiss the symptoms as trivial as, unfortunately, this is a common societal view of some invisible illnesses.

It's easy to exclaim, 'Pull yourself together!', 'All you need to do is just eat your meal!' or 'Everyone gets tired.' Sometimes, people think comments such as, 'Yes, I have had a bit of IBS too' show empathy, but you might not feel the same.

They should be assured that the symptoms are real and not to be trivialized or derided. The IBS expert is you. Education lets others know what you can cope with. Explain that the symptoms can be unpredictable and this could mean you might not always be able to go out and you may have to cancel plans you have made at the last minute.

Direct loved ones to a trusted website, such as the IBS Network (<theibsnetwork.org>), to learn more, especially if you feel uncomfortable talking about it. Education also helps change attitudes to invisible conditions.

Self-help groups

The IBS Network supports self-help groups; if you want to join one see the organization's website for details of local groups. The groups rely on volunteers to run them, so consider starting a group if one is not already established in your area.

Volunteering

Of benefit to your community – but also to you, and possibly to your IBS!

Volunteering for local initiatives can help in many ways: it can get you out of the house, offer some light exercise, combat isolation and help you make new friends, boost mood and self-confidence – all of which could have a positive effect on your IBS.

It needn't be a big commitment: volunteer for just two hours a week, if you like.

Think about what you'd like to achieve with your time – be it improve your local area, help disadvantaged people, find a new hobby, learn a new skill or make new friends.

Also think about what you have to offer and what you are willing to offer – in terms of skills, time and taking on responsibilities. Take care with this at first – you don't wish to take on board anything that will be stressful, so it's important to set clear boundaries in your mind.

Find volunteering opportunities at your local arts centres, libraries, charity shops, places of worship, social clubs, environmental or animal-care groups, sports teams, youth groups, old people's homes, hospitals and many more besides. Read noticeboards at supermarkets, newsagents and libraries, or look at local papers for openings.

Try not to commit to more than you can handle. Don't be afraid to ask questions of the supervisors at the organization you're interested in. If any difficulties arise, voice them straight away and don't let concerns fester.

Talking therapies

Self-help and help from family and acquaintances are great – but can the professionals help too?

There are many psychological therapies available and sometimes they are loosely called 'counselling' – although counselling is a therapy in its own right. Research shows these can be hugely beneficial to some with IBS when combined with dietary and other lifestyle modifications.

The basic reasoning underpinning these therapies centres on the 'dual carriageway' that is the brain–gut axis: how beliefs, emotions, thoughts and feelings impact on the gut and the intensification of gut symptoms, and how the person emotionally responds to physical symptoms experienced – for instance, by focusing too intently on them.

They are not a 'magic wand'. They don't always work well, depending on the individual, and you may need to be patient and invest effort in the treatment.

Availability through the NHS varies, so private referral may be your only viable option if it is suggested to you by your GP. That said, the situation has improved somewhat since 2010, when the government made psychological therapies more widely available via a national programme called Improved Access to Psychological Therapies (IAPT). Access to IAPT varies by region – some accept self-referrals, others will require a referral from your GP.

According to NICE guidelines, 'referral for psychological interventions should be considered for people with IBS who do not respond to pharmacological treatments after 12 months'. Chat with your GP about which of the therapies may suit you best.

Interestingly, a study published in the *American Journal of Gastroenterology* suggests that online (internet-based) therapies and stress management programmes, which would obviate the need for people to visit therapists in person, may be reasonably good substitutes – especially with younger people who are more comfortable with modern communications media. Ensure that any such programmes are developed by appropriately qualified practitioners or recommended by relevant associations (see under 'Counselling and mental health' in the Useful addresses section). For instance, the British Association for Behavioural and Cognitive Psychotherapies (BABCP) suggests 'Living Life to the Full' (www.llttf.com).

Counselling

This is a 'gentle' talking therapy.

Counsellors will listen sympathetically to you and will aim to empathize with your situation and any issues that are causing you emotional difficulties and may therefore be aggravating or triggering IBS flare-ups.

By talking and listening, they may help you to clarify issues that you're struggling with. You will be encouraged to be open with your feelings. Counsellors may offer gentle advice but will not tell you what to do: in general, their aim is to guide you to work towards solving any issues you have. They can, for instance, help those with IBS to come to terms with the impact it can have on their life.

Psychotherapy

This is a more analytical, 'deeper' talking therapy, which may be suited to those with more embedded anxieties or those who have suffered difficult experiences or past traumas that may be having an impact on their everyday lives.

A good, trusting relationship with your therapist is particularly important, and the treatment may in some cases be lengthy. It may help you to address intractable situations in new ways, however, and develop fresh coping mechanisms to accept difficulties in your life.

Cognitive behavioural therapy (CBT)

CBT is a short-term form of psychotherapy that explores your behavioural responses to thoughts and feelings – and how subsequent actions impact those feelings. It focuses on both patterns of thought (cognitions) and actions (behaviour).

It is concerned with how you handle dilemmas. It challenges negative thought patterns, helps you to identify and understand them, equips you with coping skills and implements changes that can be made to unhelpful thinking or behaviour. The therapy is structured, practical and result-focused, unlike counselling, which usually involves 'freer' conversation and a greater rapport with the therapist.

It is an active therapy. You will be given 'homework' – experimenting with thinking and acting differently – with the eventual goal of self-management.

CBT for IBS will help you see bowel symptoms as expressions of the anxiety you experience in life rather than expressions of disease. The aim of this is that it gives you more control over your symptoms and ownership and responsibility for your irritable bowel.

Hypnotherapy

This is a method, often used in psychotherapy, that uses hypnosis – a state of deep relaxation and heightened awareness, which makes the mind more receptive to positive suggestion.

Unfortunately, hypnotherapy has a 'magical' reputation due to television shows using hypnosis as entertainment. This can make individuals nervous of it, as they fear they may lose control – but this is not the case. You will not be asleep or unconscious, and will be free to move or speak. It will be a little like losing yourself in a book when reading or watching a film and being absorbed in the content.

It can help those suffering from low self-esteem and anxiety, for instance, but also helps with stress management, positive thinking and relaxation techniques.

There is good evidence that a technique called gut-directed hypnotherapy can help with IBS symptoms in about 70 per cent of people. Unfortunately, this treatment is not widely available in the NHS, but private practitioners registered with a professional body (see the Useful addresses section) can be considered.

8

Physical well-being

As well as your emotional well-being, your physical well-being needs to be looked after! With so much focus on your gut and your diet, it can be easy to neglect other areas that are necessary for maintaining good health – and because physical health can boost emotional health, it is doubly important to take these into account.

Activity and exercise

If you have any medical conditions that affect your ability to perform activities, discuss starting any activity or exercise with your doctor or physiotherapist before going ahead.

It's not a very exciting message, and we all know it already, but exercise is good for you – and it may well help to relieve symptoms of IBS. Your doctor or physiotherapist may be able to suggest the best kind for you, be it walking, jogging or swimming. Aim for two to three hours weekly at least of aerobic exercise – which increases your heart and breathing rates.

Yoga is thought to be helpful, but you may also benefit from t'ai chi or Pilates, which can be restful as well as dynamic.

If none of these appeal and you hate the gym, try to spend more time on hobbies that involve movement – gardening or amateur dramatics, for instance – rather than seated activities (online gaming, jigsaw puzzles, etc.).

Avoid sitting for too long. If you work in an office, seated at a desk for much of the day, take a five- or ten-minute break to move around every hour.

Runner's diarrhoea

We know exercise can speed up bowel transit, so it can be useful if you are constipated. Some forms of exercise can contribute to diarrhoea, however. Running may be one; the internal organs and bowel are 'jostled' more than during other activities (swimming or cycling), possibly increasing the effect. Some believe that reduced blood flow to the bowel, as it is redirected towards muscles and elsewhere, puts the bowel under extra 'stress'. Try lowering the speed and intensity of your runs if it's a continuing problem. Avoid tight leggings or vests, which can pressure the bowel.

If, despite any dietary adjustments, you still experience symptoms, try avoiding food in the hours leading up to exercise, but take liquids as dehydration can make matters worse. Take care with 'energy bars' or 'sports nutrition' products, which can be high-FODMAP foods.

Posture

Sometimes a poor or hunched posture can trigger abdominal discomfort, and this could be an area worth working on, via exercise. Here's one.

1 Lie on your back on a yoga mat, with a folded and rolled hand towel across the bottom of your shoulder blades.
2 Bend your knees, place your feet flat on the floor and position arms at your side.
3 Stretch your arms into the air above your head, then return.
4 Belly breathe through your nose and notice your upper chest muscles in neutral. Lie for two minutes, allowing spine to relax and gently extend.
5 Roll over on to hands and knees.
6 Sit back on your heels, stretching arms out in front, chin tucked in as you breathe out. Hold for ten seconds. Keep breathing!
7 Go back to hands and knees, then lie fully on your front.
8 Place your hands under your shoulders and gently lift head and shoulders, breathing in. Rest on your forearms. Breathe in and out five times and then lower yourself.
9 Roll on to your back again, with the towel under your head and legs straight.
10 Bend both knees up and clasp with your hands, pulling your knees gently up to your chest. Relax in this position, while breathing into your lower back.

11 Lower your right leg and straighten it. Place your left foot on the floor on the outside of your right knee, so your left knee is bent. Reach with your right hand to outside your bent knee and gently pull the knee to the right. Feel the outside of your hip stretch gently. Hold the stretch, breathe, then release.

12 Repeat 11 with your straight left leg and right foot on the outside of your left knee.

13 Lie fully stretched out and check for tight spots. Breathe into the tense area, and breathe out the tension. When fully relaxed, enjoy feeling loose. Take two minutes to breathe slowly, releasing and relaxing, keeping knees bent if your lower back is sore.

14 If your legs ache, raise them up a wall, with your bottom as close to the wall as possible and arms flat on the floor. Breathe slowly while relaxing.

15 Enjoy a full body stretch before rolling on to all fours to stand up slowly.

Smoking

This is hugely detrimental to health, increasing risks of cancer and heart disease.

It also has an impact on the digestive system. As it is a powerful stimulant, tobacco can worsen heartburn or reflux, and smoking can alter the sensitivity of the bowel. Some with IBS-C report that a cigarette can help them pass a motion thanks to the stimulation of tobacco, but long-term use is damaging and will only worsen digestive symptoms.

Smoking increases stress, which affects IBS. You may also nervously swallow air while you smoke and this has effects on IBS too.

There are many tools available from your doctor or pharmacy. Even if you have failed with one method, consider another. Don't be despondent if you don't succeed first time: most ex-smokers try to quit more than once. For help see NHS Smokefree (<www.nhs.uk/smokefree>).

Sleep

Although most of us occasionally have a bad night's rest, for around one in four insomnia is a more regular problem. Disturbance in sleep is associated with a less healthy microbiome and increased stress – neither good, potentially, for IBS. But if counting sheep hasn't worked for you and you don't wish to start taking sleeping tablets, what can you do?

Food . . .

There is no good evidence that certain foods can help you sleep, but some people do seem to react better or worse to particular evening meals. Experiment.

Some believe foods containing tryptophan – an amino acid needed to produce the sleep-inducing hormones serotonin and melatonin in the brain – are a wise choice before bedtime. Furthermore, eating carbohydrates with tryptophan-rich foods is thought to increase the amino acid's availability to the brain, and calcium additionally helps the production of melatonin. Although there is little evidence for this, there's no harm in trying. Poultry, meat, eggs and whole grains are high in tryptophan, as are dairy foods, soya products, beans, pulses and some nuts and seeds, which are also calcium-rich.

Avoiding late, heavy meals is important, not only because your system will be kept busy and active, with rumblings and wind, which may keep you awake, but also because it may provoke night-time heartburn or gastro-oesophageal reflux. At night, your biological clock tries to reduce body temperature in order to get it ready for sleep. A large meal just before bed starts off digestive processes that raise body temperature. This works against what your body is aiming for. The maxim 'don't dine after nine' holds true. Very fatty meals are inadvisable as well, as these add considerably to your digestive system's workload. Spicy or hot or highly seasoned food can make heartburn worse.

If late-night hunger pangs strike, try a little cereal with milk – or some peanut butter on a piece of wholegrain toast. Oats are thought to be soothing too, so oatcakes are a good light snack if you're peckish late in the evening – they give a slow release of energy that isn't too stimulating.

If you wake up hungry, again an oatcake, half a banana or a small piece of hard cheese may be all you need to fill that gap and allow you to drift back to sleep. If this is a regular occurrence, you may not be eating enough at dinner. Many women worry about eating average-sized portions for their evening meal because they believe calories consumed later in the day are less likely to be 'burned off' overnight, leading to weight gain. There is no evidence for this – it is total calorie intake during the 24-hour period that counts rather than when food is consumed.

. . . and drink

Avoiding too much alcohol is key. Although a 'nightcap' can increase drowsiness, it's not something to come to rely on or to be recommended. If you drink too much alcohol before bed, you'll experience something more like unconsciousness than sleep, and wake up unrefreshed.

Similarly, caffeine intake could be problematic.

Some people swear by hot milk to help them sleep – though choose low-lactose milk, if you need to.

For a herbal drink, try lemon verbena. Chamomile is good, but contains FODMAPs.

Interrupted sleep

Other than hunger, this may be caused by a number of issues.

Restless legs

Also known as Ekbom's Syndrome, this is characterized by tingling, twitching and discomfort in the legs and an urge to move them repeatedly in order to relieve the unpleasant feelings. Some describe an annoying 'crawling' sensation.

It can be a side effect of certain drugs and medications (such as antidepressants, antihistamines or steroids) or a sign of kidney conditions or an underactive thyroid.

Stretching, movement and massage can help relieve symptoms – both before bed and if you're woken by any occurrence of them during the night.

Some researchers believe low iron levels may be linked to restless legs, particularly in young women.

Nocturia

This is having to get up to pass water more than once during the night. Usually, especially in younger people, this happens because you've drunk too much fluid or didn't empty your bladder fully before bedtime. Yoga and Pilates or any other activity that works the pelvic floor can tighten the muscles around your bladder too, giving you the urge to pee more regularly, including at night. Other possibilities include underlying cystitis or (more rarely) an early sign of diabetes. In men, it could also be benign prostatic hyperplasia (BPH) – a natural swelling of the prostate gland, common as men age.

If it happens, just get up out of bed calmly, walk to the loo, empty your bladder and don't flush (the noise will wake you further). Don't turn on lights if you can make the journey to the bathroom safely. Avoid looking at the time, and just go back to bed.

If it happens regularly, try to plan for the event so that your journey to the loo is easy and not disruptive – leave relevant doors open and the loo seat down. Rather than drinking less total fluid during the whole day, drink more in the morning and afternoon and less late at night. Get blood sugar levels tested to ensure it's not diabetes.

Snoring

Noisy vibrations in your mouth and throat when you're asleep affect many – and many partners!

There are muscles in your throat, mouth and nose that keep airways open during the day and relax at night – this relaxation can sometimes cause these airways to close up, restricting incoming and outgoing air, making the vibrations more likely.

Snoring isn't usually a health problem unless it wakes you and disturbs your sleep or that of your partner, or if you are tired during the day and are waking up unrefreshed. Smoking, alcohol and allergies can all contribute to snoring, and if you're overweight and not having restful sleep, you may have a condition called sleep apnoea. Weight loss can help.

Over-the-counter products such as nasal strips and throat sprays are said to help by opening up and lubricating the airways. Try elevating the head of your bed or using different pillows. A eucalyptus steam inhalation can help blocked nasal passages.

Acid reflux

This is a problem for many with IBS. It can cause heartburn and is particularly troublesome at night when you're lying down.

It can be aggravated by alcohol, coffee, fatty foods and smoking. Pregnant women and the overweight are more susceptible.

Avoid heavy meals at night, and raise the head of your bed. Consider medications such as antacids. See also the advice on page 52.

Good sleep tips

If your sleep is disordered or you are waking up regularly at night, try some of the following, and some of the relaxation techniques on pages 91–3 too.

- Stick to a regular 'schedule' of sleep – going to bed and getting up at roughly the same time – to help 'set' your body clock.
- Avoid long daytime 'siestas' and limit yourself to a 15-minute cat nap at most, if you need it.
- Expose yourself to light during the day – perhaps combining it with some exercise – and ensure your home or office are well lit. Light exposure helps regulate sleep hormones.
- In the evening, avoid bright light from televisions, computers or e-readers, as well as domestic lighting.
- Also avoid too much stimulation – from your PC, television or a thrilling book. Soft music or something soothing on the radio is better.
- A 'winding down' ritual can help: a warm bath or just getting changed into pyjamas and settling down with a warm drink can be enough – something you do in a relaxed atmosphere, perhaps by candlelight.
- Your bedroom should be cooler than your living room. If you ever sweat, it may be too warm; if you're tense in bed or find yourself hiding under the covers, too cool. Aim for around 16 °C.
- Is your bedroom a bedroom – or a room for other purposes? Remove any clutter. Try to create a haven entirely focused on sleep.
- Are you comfortable in bed? Is your mattress too hard or too soft? Stiffness when you wake may indicate a problem.

- It should be dark – try an eye mask if it isn't.
- If you're bothered by something that's keeping you awake, turn the light on, write it down, set it aside and resolve to think about it tomorrow, when you are less tired.

IBS and menstruation

Some women find symptoms are worse during their period. This is due to changes in levels of hormones affecting the functioning of the muscles in the bowel and the degree of perception of pain. IBS has also been found to affect rectal sensitivity during hormone cycles and increases have been shown for all IBS symptoms.

Evidence of the effect of menopause on IBS is contradictory – some women find IBS improves, others don't. Symptoms of IBS can overlap with symptoms of endometriosis. If your level of pain is severe before and during your period, tell your doctor.

Sex

Well, it's another option if you can't sleep . . . But, seriously, your sex life can be affected by IBS, and it's a subject that we shouldn't shy away from.

Women with IBS are considerably more likely to report sexual dysfunction and painful intercourse – but men are also affected. These are hardly surprising consequences of the increased stress and abdominal discomfort that come with IBS, but pain may be due to the greater visceral hypersensitivity individuals experience, which could extend to other organs, the vagina included.

A 2013 study found that a third of women admit that their IBS has put significant pressure on their intimate relationships. Loss of libido is an obvious consequence of feeling unwell, but women who do engage in sex may feel sore and experience tummy upsets. Those with IBS-C may find sexual activity particularly uncomfortable.

Dr Barbara Bolen, an American psychotherapist who specializes in IBS, says 'intimate communication' with your partner is vital – and suggests couples counselling in situations where a long-term partner is finding it difficult to support or understand you.

Sexuality expert Cory Silverberg is also an advocate of 'outing' discussions on IBS and sex. If you fear losing control of your bladder or bowel during sex, he says, speak to your partner. He suggests that you very specifically consider what precisely you feel worried or ashamed about: that your partner might see or smell your urine or faeces? That it may ruin the moment – or the sheets? Understanding this will help you understand your expectations of what sex should be like – and help you broach the subject with your lover.

He also advises you avoid using sanitized words and terms ('having an accident') – and instead use whatever terms come naturally to you – use 'poo' (or stronger) if that's what you normally say. The point is that euphemisms keep us feeling ashamed.

Understanding that 'normal' sex is messy, and that anyone (not just those with IBS) can lose control of bodily functions during sex, can remove some of the stress.

Another tip: sex means much more than just intercourse. Explore non-penetrative forms of sex, and don't assume your partner will not be satisfied with them.

9

Practical matters

IBS can touch all aspects of your life, not only how you eat and feel, but also how you live, work and relax.

Using the bathroom

We all have to 'go' but are rarely taught how to empty our bowel properly.

It's important not to ignore a call of nature – however frequently or infrequently it comes.

A warm and comfortable toilet helps. Use a heater in colder months, or a toilet seat warmer.

Avoid straining. It's important to relax, avoid slouching or hunching, and allow yourself the time you need. Let the urge intensify, but don't force it. A gentle push to help the movement is fine, but don't 'bear down' on your bowel.

Sit on the toilet with your feet on the floor and knees higher than your hips – use a footrest if you need to. Lean forward a little, rest your elbows on your knees, bulge out your abdomen slightly and straighten your spine.

Here is a technique called the abdominal brace, devised by nurses at University College Hospital, which makes opening the bowel easier when you feel the urge.

1 Place your hands on your waist and cough. You will feel the muscles in your waist widen, and these are the muscles you should use.
2 Take a few deep breaths and slowly 'brace' outwards, widening your waist.
3 Gently push downwards from your waist towards your bottom, allowing a stool to pass.
4 Relax, then carry out the method again until your bowel is empty. Do not strain.

If the urge passes while you're sitting on the toilet, get up, carry on with your routine normally and wait for it to return.

Massage for constipation

Abdominal massage for constipation is a gentle clockwise massage over your abdomen, which can be effective. It should not be used in pregnancy or if you have another serious bowel condition. Check with a doctor first.

Here is a straightforward exercise, but there are variations that you may find online.

1 Lie on your back, preferably on your bed. Relax.
2 Place your dominant hand flat down on your abdomen and gently move it clockwise around your navel.
3 Gradually increase the pressure and expand the circle of motion until the massage is quite firm and wide, completing up to ten full circles.
4 Breathe slowly and gently throughout.

Wind

Another topic we should not shy away from is gas or 'farting'.

Those not bothered by gas may argue that it's a case of 'better out than in' – and they're right, as gas shouldn't be held in your gut, where it can cause symptoms. However, our social mores mean few of us have the freedom to not care about passing wind.

At work, take a toilet break or leave the office if you can, where you can 'safely' release any gas. If you need to pass wind in a public toilet and are hesitant, use a cubicle and employ a 'courtesy flush' to mask any sounds.

If the wind is smelly, ventilate the cubicle or room if you can, and try neutralizing products such as the Auricare Odour Eliminator or those by Neutradol, other air fresheners or simply striking a match.

Wind-deodorizing underwear (such as Shreddies) is also available.

'Going' away from home

Most of us would prefer the comfort of a home loo, but this isn't always practical – friends' loos, public toilets and the facilities at work will all need to be used!

If you're uncomfortable using unfamiliar loos, use disinfectant wipes to clean the seat and use a portable loo seat cover.

For odour, try Happy Flush.

The website The Great British Public Toilet Map (<https://great-britishpublictoiletmap.rca.ac.uk/>) can help you locate a loo if you're struggling.

Some public toilets are kept locked and may be fitted with National Key Scheme (NKS) locks. A key to open them – called a radar key – can be bought by people with a recognized disability or health condition that might mean toilet access is required. It is available from the IBS Network and Disability Rights UK (see Useful addresses section).

The IBS Network has 'Can't Wait' cards, which you can present in a shop or other establishment if you have a sudden need for a bathroom. Although not a guarantee, they are widely recognized and people are likely to help if you're caught short. The charity also sells an emergency toilet kit that contains a freshener, hand gel, 'Can't Wait' card, tissues and a self-dampened cloth, which it can be useful to keep in your bag.

Essentials checklist

Here are some key items that may come in handy when you're away from home (see the Useful addresses section for contact details and outlets):

- 'Can't Wait' card
- radar key
- digestive enzymes – see page 61 (useful to take with you when eating away from home if you're concerned about FODMAPs)
- air freshener
- hand gel
- wet wipes or portable toilet rolls
- incontinence items
- spare underwear and bags
- antidiarrhoea tablets, rehydration salts, bottled water
- phone numbers – of IBS Network, your healthcare providers and others.

Travel

Holidaying and travelling can be a daunting prospect.

Sitting for extended periods on journeys, such as long-haul flights, can make constipation worse. Having diarrhoea, with its associated difficulties of finding available toilets in unfamiliar or restricted surroundings, may cause anxiety. Many choose to stay close to home because of it.

Anecdotally, however, many find their symptoms ease on holiday, so is the aggravation of travel worth it for the 'reward' of relief when you arrive?

Planning

Prepare! Do as much as you can, as soon as you can, so you don't feel rushed or stressed as departure day looms.

If you have dietary restrictions, choose a destination the cuisines of which are likely to suit you. Much Japanese food is naturally low FODMAP and the food of south-east Asia is largely gluten- and dairy-free. That said, awareness of the gluten-free diet is growing in Europe, so you should easily find wheat-free products in countries such as Italy – though be wary of onion and garlic.

Before you book, explain the situation to your travel operator, and research hotels in advance – particularly their catering facilities. Hotels with a fridge in the room (allowing you to store safe snacks) can help, but you may wish to self-cater if your diet is complex. If you suffer from food intolerances, contact the airline to book in-flight meals in advance.

Work within your symptoms – if they are worse at a particular time of day, travel outside that time. Book seats in advance, as near to the toilet as you feel comfortable, preferably an aisle seat, and research facilities at airports and train stations.

Don't plan to do too much during your vacation – less is more! You are more likely to enjoy the experience if you choose one or two excursions rather than pack your itinerary.

Setting out

If you follow the low-FODMAP diet, strictly avoid any foods that result in symptoms for at least 48 hours before you leave.

Take spare clothing, deodorizers, wet wipes or the IBS Network's emergency kit in your hand luggage – bearing in mind fluid restrictions on flights (<www.gov.uk/hand-luggage-restrictions>).

Leave plenty of time to get to the airport or to your destination if staying in the UK. Don't rush: try to use travelling as part of the holiday experience. It doesn't matter if it takes longer to arrive: sometimes, minor roads are a great alternative to motorways. Research and plan toilet stops along the route.

You can use a 'Can't Wait' card on a plane. Explain your situation to a flight assistant: you don't need to go into details, and can just say that you have a medical condition that may require urgent toilet use.

Staying symptom-free

Get up and move around, if you can, during your flight or train journey as this helps to release trapped gas – and cuts the risk of blood clots!

Flying can lead to gas in the colon expanding and this might potentially make symptoms of bloating worse. Avoid sparkling drinks.

If you have pre-arranged an in-flight meal, confirm that it is correct when it arrives.

If you suffer from motion sickness, choose a cabin or seat in the middle of the boat or plane and use a headrest to keep your head still. Motion sickness often occurs when your eyes see movement and this is not matched by the balance sensors in your ears, confusing your brain. Look at a still object such as the horizon, or close your eyes. Reading can make symptoms worse. See a GP or pharmacist before you travel as medication can help.

At your destination

Toilet facilities abroad may be different from what you are used to at home. Keep spare change in the local currency to quickly access public toilets.

Consider hiring a car and driving around – that way, you're in control of your own stops.

'Can't Wait' cards from the IBS Network are available in other languages – don't be shy of using yours if you need to! Translation

Table 9.1 Translations of basic terms

English	French	German	Italian	Spanish
Without onion	Sans oignon	Ohne zwiebel	Senza cipolla	Sin cebolla
Without garlic	Sans ail	Ohne knoblauch	Senza aglio	Sin ajo
Gluten-free	Sans gluten	Ohne gluten	Senza glutine	Sin gluten
Wheat-free	Sans blé	Ohne weizen	Senza grano	Sin trigo

cards, with expressions useful in finding toilets abroad, come with membership. You can get travel cards online for dietary needs. Table 9.1 gives some basic terms translated into the four major European languages.

Carry rehydration salts in your first aid pack, in case you get diarrhoea, and doubly so if holidaying in a hot climate. Eight to ten glasses of fluids are usually adequate but dark urine is a sign you need more.

Obviously, follow commonsense hygiene advice. Wash hands religiously, stick to bottled water, and if you're uncertain about hygiene, opt for cooked foods rather than raw (such as salads). The last thing you want is a case of traveller's diarrhoea.

10

Moving forward

You may be wondering what the future holds – both for you, and for IBS.

Your continuing health

You may, understandably, be worried about the future – both managing your symptoms in the long term, and the thought of having to live with them for the rest of your life.

IBS symptoms can come and go, and there will be times when your symptoms are less severe and times when you are experiencing a flare-up. The way to manage is to understand what your symptoms are and try treatments specifically for them. Not all will work, but it is important to try.

Henry Ford, founder of the car company named after him, said: 'if you think you can, or you think you can't – you're right.' In essence: adopting a positive attitude to treatments can be beneficial.

Realize that failure of a treatment never reflects a failure on your part; *no* treatment for *any* medical condition is universally effective. If you focus on the symptom you would most like to address, and tackle one at a time, you'll better understand which treatment helps which symptom. In practice, some will require more than one.

Severe symptoms

There may be times when pain is severe and you wonder whether it can possibly be IBS or something more serious. This situation shouldn't stop you from trying treatments.

You will, over time, become aware of what your usual symptoms are, and if these change in any way then this is the time to discuss with your doctor. Any 'red flag' changes must be referred to your GP.

GP review

The NICE quality standards for IBS suggest that you agree follow-up care with your GP and schedule an annual review, if appropriate – either in person at the practice, or by telephone.

Medical research

It is a progressive time. We are seeing a great deal of research – the IBS Network updates its members on this via its magazine, *Gut Reaction* – and IBS feels less of a 'Cinderella' condition than it did before. We have a way to go before it is less stigmatized and marginalized, but can be confident that improvements in treatments will come.

Testing for IBS after gastrointestinal infection

A new test was developed in the United States in 2015. Called IBSchek, it looks for antibodies to both CdtB – a toxin produced by gastroenteritis-causing bacteria – and vinculin – a protein that lines the gut. Antibodies to CdtB also react with vinculin, which, it is proposed, causes damage to the gut lining, leading to the key symptoms of IBS.

Researchers have found the test distinguishes patients with IBS from those with inflammatory bowel disorders, thereby helping to confirm diagnosis.

This test is only available privately in the UK at present and would probably need approval from health bodies ahead of future use within the NHS. Because the test only identifies IBS-D after a gastrointestinal infection, it may only be useful for a subset of people with IBS.

Faecal microbiota transplantation (FMT)

This is the transplantation of a sample of stool from a healthy individual into the bowel of a patient with digestive complaints for therapeutic purposes. It is commonly termed a poo transplant!

FMT is not a new idea. It has been used for such conditions as resistant infections of *Clostridium difficile* – a particularly nasty bacterial pathogen – for which it has impressive (90 per cent) effectiveness.

Now it is also being researched in other digestive conditions where a disordered microbiome is possibly involved – such as IBS.

Should this treatment become available, it must only be considered through the NHS, for which it will have been carefully vetted and approved. There are some private availability and 'home treatment' recommendations online, but this is categorically *not* something to self-administer or undergo without strict protocols having been followed. Much more research is needed, but it is promising.

Zonulin

People with IBS and non-coeliac gluten sensitivity have higher levels of a protein called zonulin in the gut.

There is a theory that pathogenic microbes can trigger the release of zonulin. The protein regulates the tight junctions between the cells lining the digestive tract. Increased zonulin means the tight junctions are 'loosened', potentially allowing larger protein molecules into the body – this is sometimes dubbed 'leaky gut'. It is speculated that this can trigger inflammation and immune system responses.

More research is needed, but drugs to control the production of zonulin may offer future potential to treat the gut lining and improve tolerance to food.

Dietary treatment

We expect the low-FODMAP diet to become more widely known – and accordingly easier to manage. More low-FODMAP food brands (a few are listed in the Useful addresses section) and low-FODMAP menus and food outlets are all expected.

A final word . . .

We hope you have found some useful advice in this book, wish you well for the future, and hope your gut gives you some peace!

Appendix 1
Food and symptom diary

Example template

Here is an example of a food and symptom diary that you can copy out to fill in or adapt as required.

Date			
Time	Food	Drink	Comments (symptoms, medication, for example)
Early morning			
Breakfast			
Mid-morning			
Lunch			
Mid-afternoon			
Evening meal			
During evening			
Supper			
Extras			

Example of a completed diary entry

Date: Monday 18 June			
Time	Food	Drink	Comments, (symptoms, medication, for example)
Early morning		One cup of tea with semi-skimmed milk	Headache 7.00 a.m., diarrhoea
Breakfast	30 g of Kellogg's cornflakes ½ cup of semi-skimmed milk Slice of wholemeal toast with margarine	200 ml glass orange juice	
Mid-morning	Three pieces of sugar-free gum		Diarrhoea 11.30
Lunch	Two slices of supermarket's own brand wholemeal bread with margarine (thinly spread), cheese and three slices tomato	Cup of tea with semi-skimmed milk and one teaspoon of white sugar	Diarrhoea 12.40 Abdominal pain 12.40
Mid-afternoon	Nakd Cashew cookie bar	Cup of tea	Abdominal pain, slight bloating
Evening meal	Tuna pasta bake (home-made) Two slices of garlic bread	One glass red wine	As above
During evening		Two cups of tea	
Supper	Two Jacob's cream crackers with Cheddar cheese		Abdominal pain, severe bloating, diarrhoea
Extras	None		

A week's worth of diary is usually adequate to assess symptoms – the more detail the better. Here are some specific points to note:

- portion sizes
- brand or manufacturer's name
- product names (precisely and in full)
- type of milk – full-fat, semi-skimmed, skimmed, UHT, plant alternative, fortified and so on
- potato – freshly cooked, oven chips, boiled, roasted, baked, fried and so on.

To review a food diary, look for symptoms associated with certain foods and any repeat of this pattern with the same food. If a food gives symptoms on one day but not another, was the portion size different? Might it have been a different ingredient? It is not often that a food will result in symptoms immediately unless it is high in fat. It might be the food you ate in the meal before or sometimes the day before.

Analysing an IBS food diary is tricky as so many different food reactions can take place. Your dietitian can help.

Appendix 2
Recipes

Here is a small selection. Other books (see page 135) will provide you with more options.

Breakfasts

Crumpets

(Makes about 10)
300 g (10½ oz) gluten-free self-raising flour
1 tsp dried yeast
2 eggs (at room temperature), beaten
445 ml (¾ pt) lactose-free milk, lukewarm
salt and pepper
spray oil, for cooking

Preheat oven to 190 °C (375 °F, gas mark 5). Combine all ingredients, mix well and leave in a warm place for yeast to act until the mix rises or bubbles (about 15 minutes). Spray a frying pan with oil and heat. Place an oil-sprayed cooking ring in the centre of the pan. Fill ring with 1 cm (just under ½ in) thickness of batter and cook for 2–3 minutes.

Lift ring, turn crumpet and cook for another 2–3 minutes. Place on a baking tray and bake in the preheated oven for 10 minutes to complete cooking.

French Toast

(Serves 2–3)

2 eggs
70 ml (2½ fl oz) lactose-free milk
4 drops vanilla essence
4 drops orange essence
2–3 slices gluten-free bread
spray oil, to cook
some mixed berries, to serve
maple syrup (or sweetener such as stevia or sucralose)

Crack eggs into a bowl and mix with milk and essences. Soak bread slices fully in egg mix (1–2 minutes). Lightly spray a frying pan with oil and fry bread for 1 minute each side or until golden. Serve warm with berries and a drizzle of syrup.

Lunches

Kale and Herb Frittata

(Serves 2–3)

handful kale
4 eggs
salt and pepper
2–3 sprigs fresh thyme or a few rosemary leaves, chopped, or pinch dried thyme
spray oil, to cook
25 g (¾–1 oz) Parmesan, grated
1 tbsp pine nuts

Boil kale until just soft. Leave to cool then chop well. Crack eggs into a bowl. Mix, season and divide into two equal portions. Add kale and herbs to one portion and mix well. Spray a little oil into a frying pan, heat, add egg and kale mix, flatten with a fork and cook for 1–2 minutes or until set. Add second egg portion and cook for 2–3 minutes. Meanwhile, heat the grill. Remove pan from heat and place under the grill to continue cooking. When eggs are risen and fluffy, sprinkle with cheese and pine nuts. Grill until cheese is melted and pine nuts are toasted.

Pumpkin Soup

(Serves 3–4)

garlic-infused oil
1 tsp coriander seeds
2-cm (¾-in) piece fresh ginger, peeled and grated
½ tsp asafoetida
½ tsp chilli powder (if tolerated)
half small pumpkin, peeled and chopped into small pieces
half small swede, peeled and chopped into small pieces
1 litre (1¾ pt) water (more if needed)

Add oil to a pan, heat, add the spices and fry for a few seconds. Add chopped vegetables with water and cook until soft. Blend until smooth.

Cheese Soufflé

(Serves 4)

olive oil
4 eggs
20 g (¾ oz) margarine
20 g (¾ oz) gluten-free plain flour or cornflour
250 ml (½ pt) lactose-free milk
pepper
170 g (6 oz) Cheddar cheese (lactose-free if you are very sensitive)

Oil eight ramekins and preheat oven to 220 °C (425 °F, gas mark 7). Carefully separate egg yolks from the whites – the whites must be free of any yolk. Melt margarine gently in a pan, add flour and stir well – this will thicken. Cook for a few seconds and slowly incorporate milk until it makes a smooth sauce. Simmer to cook the flour, stirring all the time. Sieve sauce if lumpy. Cool slightly and add yolks, stirring well. Season with some pepper and melt in the cheese. Whisk egg whites until they form stiff peaks. Add a third of the egg whites to the sauce to slacken it, then fold the rest into the sauce carefully until fully incorporated – stop immediately this point is reached as you need as much air as possible in the mix. Divide the mixture between the ramekins and cook in the preheated oven for about 12 minutes, until well risen and set. Serve at once.

Potato and Mackerel Soup

(Serves 2–3)

1 tbsp garlic-infused oil
asafoetida
800 g (1 lb 12 oz) potatoes, peeled and diced
1 carrot, chopped
1½ smoked mackerel fillets, flaked
300 ml (½ pt) lactose-free milk
1 litre (1¾ pt) water
salt and pepper
nutmeg

Add oil to a large pan, add a sprinkling of asafoetida and fry for a few seconds. Add vegetables and mackerel and fry gently for 2 minutes. Add milk and water, bring to the boil and simmer until vegetables are soft. Add salt and pepper to taste. Blend or mash as preferred, and finish with a grating of nutmeg.

Quinoa Salad

(Serves 2–3)

½ tsp smoked paprika
½ tsp cinnamon
¼ tsp ginger
1 dsp garlic-infused oil
25 g (¾–1 oz) sunflower and pumpkin seeds
25 g (¾–1 oz) chopped walnuts
25 g (¾–1 oz) pine nuts
1 red pepper
2 carrots
spray oil
150 g (5 oz) red quinoa
juice of half a lemon

Preheat oven to 200 °C (400 °F, gas mark 6). Add spices to garlic-infused oil and mix in the nuts and seeds. Spread in a single layer on a baking sheet and toast for 5–10 minutes in the oven – watch this closely as it can easily burn. Remove from oven and cool. Chop the pepper and carrots, spray with oil and roast in the oven for 20 minutes. Cool. Put quinoa in a pan with water to cover and simmer until soft (about 15 minutes). Cool and drain off the water. Mix with the nuts, seeds and vegetables, and add lemon juice.

Chicken Rice Salad

(Serves 3)

150 g (5 oz) brown basmati rice
30 g (1 oz) wild rice
20 g (¾ oz) Camargue red rice
1 tbsp garlic-infused oil
15 g (½ oz) fresh tarragon
2 chicken (or turkey) breasts, cooked
1 tbsp light mayonnaise or mayonnaise alternative
1 tbsp gluten-free wholegrain mustard
40 g (1½ oz) pine nuts
5 radishes, sliced
5-cm (2-in) piece cucumber, chopped
salt and pepper

Add the rices to a pan with water and simmer until cooked (about 40 minutes). Drain. Add oil and tarragon to warm rice in a bowl and mix. Chop meat and add. Chill in the fridge for 15 minutes. Combine the mayonnaise and mustard and add to the rice with pine nuts, sliced radishes and chopped cucumber. Mix thoroughly. Add salt and pepper to taste.

Evening meals

Turkey Burgers

(Serves 5–6)

600 g (1 lb 5 oz) turkey mince
1 egg, beaten
2 small carrots, grated
10 g (¼–½ oz) fresh coriander leaves, chopped
2 tsp ground coriander
1 tsp chilli powder (optional)
2.5-cm (1-in) piece fresh ginger, peeled and grated
1 tsp cumin
½ level tsp asafoetida
salt and pepper

Preheat oven to 200 °C (400 °F, gas mark 6) or preheat grill. Combine all ingredients in a bowl and mix well. Spoon a tablespoon of the mix into a dry frying pan and cook for 1–2 minutes each side until browned, repeating until all mix is cooked. Finish off in oven or grill until thoroughly cooked through.

Potato and Salmon Rosti

(Serves 2)

2 small salmon steaks
1 large potato, grated
1 egg, beaten
salt and pepper

For the green salad
alfalfa
cucumber, finely chopped

Preheat oven to 200 °C (400 °F, gas mark 6). Grill salmon steaks, allow to cool and flake. Add to the potato and bind using egg. Season with salt and pepper. Drop spoonfuls of the mixture on to a greased baking tray and cook in the preheated oven for 15 minutes. Serve with the fresh green salad.

Thai Pork Loin

(Serves 4)

1 pork tenderloin, trimmed and cut into strips
2 star anise
2.5-cm (1-in) piece fresh ginger, peeled and grated
1 tbsp low-fat peanut butter
1 tbsp garlic-infused oil
1 tbsp tamari soy sauce
15 g (½ oz) fresh coriander
100 ml (3½ fl oz) stock (home-made, vegetable or pork)
juice of ½ lime
salt
2 carrots, peeled and cut into strips with a potato peeler
3 pak choi, sliced
sesame seeds to decorate
boiled rice, to serve

Put tenderloin strips in a dish. Blend star anise, grated ginger, peanut butter, oil, soy sauce, coriander and stock, and pour resulting sauce over the pork. Add lime juice and salt and leave to marinate for at least two hours. Cook the pork mix and sauce in a pan until tender. Transfer to a wok, add carrots and pak choi and cook until the vegetables are *al dente*. Remove star anise before serving. Sprinkle with sesame seeds and serve with boiled rice.

Stir-fry Beef

(Serves 3)

2.5-cm (1-in) piece fresh ginger, peeled and grated
1 tbsp golden syrup
1 tbsp garlic-infused oil
250 g (9 oz) lean beef, cut into strips
1 spring onion, green part only, chopped
4 tbsp tamari soy sauce
1 pak choi
1 courgette, thinly sliced
1 red pepper, thinly sliced
½ x 225-g tin bamboo shoots, drained
boiled rice, to serve

Put ginger, syrup and oil in a mortar and pestle and grind to a paste. Add this to the beef and chopped spring onion, pour on soy sauce, mix well and leave to marinate for at least 30 minutes. Add beef and marinade to a heated wok, add remaining vegetables and stir-fry until cooked. Serve with boiled rice.

Fish Cakes

(Serves 4–6)

650 g (1 lb 7 oz) new potatoes
pepper
9 g (¼ oz) fresh turmeric
1 tbsp garlic-flavoured oil
2 tsp cumin
300 g (10½ oz) white fish, poached and flaked
2 eggs, beaten
150 g (5 oz) wheat-free breadcrumbs
spray oil

Preheat oven to 200 °C (400 °F, gas mark 6). Boil potatoes until soft, leaving some unpeeled for added fibre, then mash with some pepper. Peel and chop turmeric and fry in oil with cumin. Add fish, and cook lightly. Combine fish and potato, and mix gently to ensure pieces of fish remain a good size. Shape by filling a small baking ring with fish and potato mix, then push out the cake. (Or shape 2 tablespoons of mix into a fish cake by hand.) Coat each fish cake with egg, then roll in breadcrumbs. Lightly fry with spray oil to brown and then finish cooking in the preheated oven for 10 minutes.

Sage and Parsnip Gnocchi

(Serves 2)

500 g (1 lb) parsnips
80 g (2¾ oz) gluten-free flour
1 tbsp sage leaves, chopped
asafoetida
1 tbsp garlic-infused olive oil
20 g (¾ oz) Parmesan cheese, grated

Wash, peel and boil parsnips in salted water until soft. Mash well. Add flour and mix well. Turn on to a floured surface and divide into four equal amounts. Roll each into a sausage shape and cut into even-sized discs. Roll each disc into a ball, then squash flat with a fork. Bring a pan of water to the boil and add a few gnocchi at a time. They will float when cooked – remove them and drain. Fry sage and a sprinkling of asafoetida in olive oil and mix with cooked gnocchi. Sprinkle over grated Parmesan to serve.

Stuffed Aubergines

(Serves 2–4)

4 aubergines
salt and pepper
olive oil
1 tsp coriander seeds
juice of ½ lemon, plus 8 lemon slices for decoration
1 tsp peanut butter
20 g (¾ oz) pumpkin seeds
25 g (¾–1 oz) red-skinned peanuts
60 g (2 oz) corn couscous
50 g (1¾ oz) low-fat hard cheese, grated
green salad, to serve

Preheat oven to 200 °C (400 °F, gas mark 6). Slice aubergines length-ways, season, and rub surface with a little olive oil. Roast in the preheated oven for 20–30 minutes. Leave the oven on, but let the aubergines cool. Remove flesh carefully, keeping skins intact and put them to one side. Mash flesh with the remaining ingredients except the cheese and salad. Distribute the mixture evenly to fill the auber-gine skins. Sprinkle with cheese. Bake in the preheated oven for 20 minutes or until the cheese has melted. Serve with fresh green salad.

Baba Ganoush

(Serves 2)

1 aubergine
1 tbsp lactose-free light mayonnaise
¼ tsp cinnamon
1 tsp cumin powder
salt
a little lactose-free yogurt
a few pine nuts, toasted
low-FODMAP crackers and olives, to serve

Preheat oven to 200 °C (400 °F, gas mark 6) and roast aubergine whole until soft (about 45 minutes, depending on size). Leave to cool. Remove skin and add flesh to a bowl together with mayonnaise, spices and a little salt. Blend until smooth. Top with lactose-free yogurt and pine nuts. Serve with low-FODMAP crackers and olives.

Useful addresses

Health charities

Coeliac UK
Third Floor
Apollo Centre
Desborough Road
High Wycombe
Buckinghamshire HP11 2QW
Tel: 01494 437278; 0333 332 2033 (helpline)
Website: www.coeliac.org.uk

Core (gut, liver and pancreas)
3 St Andrews Place
London NW1 4LB
Tel: 020 7486 0341
Website: www.corecharity.org.uk

Disability Rights UK
Ground Floor
CAN Mezzanine
49–51 East Road
London N1 6AH
Tel: 020 7250 8181
Website: www.disabilityrightsuk.org
Radar key information: www.disabilityrightsuk.org/shop/radar-key

Endometriosis UK
Suites 1 & 2
46 Manchester Street
London W1U 7LS
Tel: 020 7222 2781; 0808 808 2227 (helpline)
Website: www.endometriosis-uk.org

The IBS Network
Unit 1.16 SOAR Works
14 Knutton Road
Sheffield S5 9NU
Tel: 0114 272 3253 (helpline available to members)
Website: www.theibsnetwork.org (IBS Self-Care Programme:
www.theibsnetwork.org/the-self-care-programme)

International organizations

Canadian Society of Intestinal Research: www.badgut.org
Coeliac Society of Ireland: www.coeliac.ie
International Foundation for Functional Gastrointestinal Disorders: www.aboutibs.org
Rome Foundation: www.theromefoundation.org

Counselling and mental health societies and associations

British Association for Behavioural and Cognitive Psychotherapies (BABCP): www.babcp.com (offers a searchable register of officially accredited CBT therapists).

British Association for Counselling and Psychotherapy (BACP): www.bacp.co.uk (see the Association's register for approved therapists at: www.bacpregister.org.uk).

British Society of Clinical and Academic Hypnosis (BSCAH): www.bscah.co.uk

National Counselling Society: www.nationalcounsellingsociety.org (offers a search facility for finding a registered and qualified counsellor in your area).

UK Council for Psychotherapy (UKCP): www.ukcp.org.uk (holds a register of psychotherapists and psychotherapeutic counsellors).

Counselling and mental health charities

Anxiety UK
Zion Community Centre
339 Stretford Road
Hulme
Manchester M15 4ZY
Tel: 08444 775 774 (infoline)
Website: www.anxietyuk.org.uk

Beat (eating disorders)
Unit 1
Chalk Hill House
19 Rosary Road
Norwich
Norfolk NR1 1SZ
Tel: 0808 801 067 (adult helpline); 0808 801 0711 (youthline)
Website: www.b-eat.co.uk

Mind (mental health)
15–19 Broadway
Stratford
London E15 4BQ
Tel: 0300 123 3393 (infoline)
Website: www.mind.org.uk

Samaritans (24-hour emotional support)
Freepost RSRB-KKBY-CYJK
PO Box 9090
Stirling FK8 2SA
Tel: 116 123 (helpline: UK or ROI)
Website: www.samaritans.org

Health and dietetic resources

BDA Freelance Dietitians Group: www.freelancedietitians.org (for help finding a FODMAP-trained dietitian).

British Dietetic Association (BDA): www.bda.uk.com

Drink Aware: www.drinkaware.co.uk

Kashrut London Beth Din: www.kosher.org.uk/koshersearch (offers a search facility for the pareve status of foods).

King's College London, FODMAPs information: www.kcl.ac.uk/fodmaps (KCL is the centre of FODMAP training and research in the UK and its website includes a regularly updated list of KCL FODMAP-trained dietitians and other information).

Manchester Beth Din: www.mbd.org.uk/site/kosher-products

Monash University, information on low-FODMAP diet for IBS: www.med. monash.edu.au/cecs/gastro/FODMAP (access this large resource at the university where researchers developed the low-FODMAP diet for a wealth of information on IBS, the diet and the university's app and certification programme).

NHS Choices weight loss guide: (www.nhs.uk/LiveWell/weight-loss-guide/ Pages/weight-loss-guide.aspx)

NHS Smokefree: www.nhs.uk/smokefree

Real Bread Campaign: www.sustainweb.org/realbread

Vegan Society: www.vegansociety.com

Vegetarian Society: www.vegsoc.org

'Free from' and low-FODMAP brands

Not all products by all brands will be suitable, but these companies' foods are worth exploring. Always check labels.

Alpro: www.alpro.com/uk (soya milk, yogurt and dessert alternatives).

BFree Foods: www.bfreefoods.co.uk (gluten-free and vegan breads, wraps and rolls).

Biona: www.biona.co.uk (gluten-free breads, rice cakes and other baked goods).

Delicious Alchemy: www.deliciousalchemy.co.uk (gluten-free bakery mixes, cereals).

Doves Farm: www.dovesfarm.co.uk (gluten-free pastas, flours, baked goods, cereals).

Eskal Foods: www.eskalfoods.com (gluten- and dairy-free pretzels, pastas, crackers and ice-cream cones).

Fodify Foods: www.fodify.co.uk (low-FODMAP savoury sauces and spice mixes).

Fodmapped (Australia): www.fodmapped.com (sauces, soups and stocks).

FODY Food Co.: www.fodyfoods.com (bouillon cubes, spice blends, protein bars, sauces and trail mixes).

General Dietary: www.generaldietary.com (gluten-free Ener-G brand pastas, baked goods, snacks, crackers).

Genius Foods: www.geniusglutenfree.com (gluten-free breads, rolls and bagels).

Glebe Farm: www.glebefarmfoods.co.uk (gluten-free flours, cakes, mixes).

Gluten Free Foods: www.glutenfree-foods.co.uk (Barkat-brand breads, pasta, flour mixes, snacks, biscuits, cakes, cereals and matzo crackers).

Hale & Hearty: www.halenhearty.co.uk (sweet and savoury mixes, cereals, pastas, snacks).

Just Milk: www.justmilk.com (low-lactose UHT milk).

Kelkin (ROI): www.kelkin.ie (bakery, cereal, pasta).

Koko Dairy Free: www.kokodairyfree.com (coconut milk, butter and yogurt alternatives).

Lactofree: www.arlafoods.co.uk/lactofree (milks, cream, spread, cheeses and yogurt, all low in lactose).

Lauren Loves: www.laurenloves.co.uk (low-FODMAP tomato sauces and infused oils).

Nairns: www.nairns-oatcakes.com (oat bakery and cereals).

Newburn Bakehouse, by Warburtons: http://www.newburnbakehouse.com (bakery and breads).

Oatly: www.oatly.co.uk (oat milks and cream).

Orgran: www.orgranglutenfree.co.uk (pasta, crispbreads, cereals, biscuits, soups, snacks, bread and flour mixes).

Provamel: www.provamel.com/uk (soya, rice and nut milk, yogurt and dessert alternatives).

Rizopia: www.rizopia.co.uk (rice pastas).

Rude Health: www.rudehealth.com (vegan milks, crackers, gluten-free cereals).

Schär: www.schaer.com/en-uk (gluten-free breads and crackers, flour, ready meals).

Slightly Different Foods: www.slightlydifferentfoods.co.uk (low-FODMAP retail suppliers and catering).

SOME Foods (Australia): www.somefoods.com.au (cooking sauces and spice mixes).

Vegusto: www.vegusto.co.uk (milk-free cheese alternatives and other vegan foods).

'Free from' online

If you can't find products in your local shops, often they will be available online, via supermarkets or specialist suppliers. Many allow you to filter by allergen or 'free from' requirement.

Amazon: www.amazon.co.uk
Free From Market: www.freefrommarket.co.uk
Goodness Direct: www.goodnessdirect.co.uk
Holland and Barrett: www.hollandandbarrett.com/info/free-from
Ocado: www.ocado.com

Sundries

Bladder & Bowel UK: www.bladderandboweluk.co.uk/products
Happy Flush (bathroom freshener): www.happyflush.com
Shreddies ('flatulence filtering underwear'): www.myshreddies.com
Value Incontinence: www.valueincontinence.co.uk

Apps

FoodMaestro FODMAP app: www.foodmaestro.me/fodmap-app (a facility to scan products to check suitability for the low-FODMAP diet in the UK. The app also helps track symptoms and is particularly useful during reintroduction. Use only with dietetic help. Available from the Apple App Store and Google Play. FoodMaestro also has an app for other dietary restrictions, such as food allergies, veganism, coeliac disease and so on).
Monash Low FODMAP Diet app: www.med.monash.edu.au/cecs/gastro/fodmap/iphone-app.html (designed primarily for the Australian diet, available from the Apple App Store and Google Play).
My Fitness Pal app: www.myfitnesspal.com (free calorie counter, available from the Apple App Store and Google Play).

Events

The Allergy and Free From Show: www.allergyshow.co.uk (annually in London, Liverpool and Glasgow).
The IBS Network conferences and events: www.theibsnetwork.org/news/events (available to members).

Further reading

Books

Arroll, Megan and Dancey, Christine (2016) *Irritable Bowel Syndrome: Navigating your way to recovery*. London: Hammersmith Health Books.

Bolen, Barbara (2015) *IBS: 365 tips for living well*. New York: Demos Health.

Gazzola, Alex (2015) *Coeliac Disease: What you need to know*. London: Sheldon Press.

Gazzola, Alex (2005) *Living with Food Intolerance*. London: Sheldon Press.

KLBD (2017) *Really Jewish Food Guide 2017/5777*. London: United Synagogue and KLBD.

Lomer, Miranda (2015) *Advanced Nutrition and Dietetics in Gastroenterology*. Hoboken, New Jersey: Wiley-Blackwell.

Ransley, Joan and Read, Nick (2016) *Cooking for the Sensitive Gut*. London: Pavilion.

Shepherd, Sue and Gibson, Peter (2014) *The Complete Low-FODMAP Diet*. London: Vermillion.

Skypala, Isabel and Venter, Carina (2009) *Food Hypersensitivity*. Hoboken, New Jersey: Wiley-Blackwell.

Blogs

Allergy Insight (Alex's Blog): www.allergy-insight.com

Clinical Alimentary (Julie's Blog): www.clinicalalimentary.wordpress.com

IBS Impact: https://ibsimpact.wordpress.com

Monash University Low FODMAP Diet: http://fodmapmonash.blogspot.co.uk

The Sensitive Gut: www.thesensitivegut.com

Websites

IBS-Free at Last!: www.ibsfree.net

IrritableBowelSyndrome.net: www.irritablebowelsyndrome.net

For a Digestive Peace of Mind, Kate Scarlata RDN: www.katescarlata.com

King's College London, FODMAPs: www.kcl.ac.uk/fodmaps

NHS Choices (IBS pages): www.nhs.uk/conditions/irritable-bowel-syndrome/Pages/Introduction.aspx

NICE (IBS guidance): www.nice.org.uk/guidance/CG61

Physiotherapy for Hyperventilation: www.physiohypervent.org

Shepherd Works: www.shepherdworks.com.au

The Great British Public Toilet Map: https://greatbritishpublictoiletmap.rca.ac.uk/

Forums

HealthUnlocked (The IBS Network's forum): https://healthunlocked.com/
theibsnetwork

Irritable Bowel Syndrome Self Help and Support Group: www.ibsgroup.org

talkibsforum (Talk Health Partnership): www.talkhealthpartnership.com/
forum/viewforum.php?f=463

Index

acid reflux 8, 16, 19, 52, 105
alcohol 8, 85–6, 103
anxiety 90, 131

bacteria, gut *see* microbiome
belching 7
bile acid malabsorption 17
biofeedback training 26
bloating 9, 26, 30–1, 34, 36, 61
blood tests 14
body mass index (BMI) 29
bowel: emptying 108–10; large 6; small 5
brain–gut axis xiv–xvi, 96
bread 28, 30, 44, 58, 72
breath tests 18, 19
breathing 88–9
Bristol Stool Form Scale 12

caffeine 30, 31–2, 36, 103
candida diet 64
carbohydrates 2, 28, 33, 42, 44
Caribbean food 79
chewing gum 9, 36, 73
Codex wheat starch 72
coeliac disease xiii, 14, 16, 57, 73, 74, 130
Coeliac UK 70, 74, 84, 130
coffee 30, 31–2, 45, 105
cognitive behavioural therapy (CBT) 97, 131
constipation 9–10, 26, 30, 34, 50–1, 109
cooking 81–2, 120–9
counselling 96–7, 131

dairy foods 28, 44; *see also* diet, dairy-free; food, dairy-free; 'free from' foods
detox diet 65
diarrhoea 7, 9, 17, 26, 29–30, 32, 46, 50, 60, 99
diet 27–8; dairy-free 58–9; *see also* 'free from' foods
diets *see under individual names*
dietitians 38–9, 42, 132
digestion xv, 1, 3–10
digestive system 4
disaccharides 42, 46, 54

eating out 82–7
elimination diet 41, 43
elimination phase (of low-FODMAP diet) 47–8
endometriosis 15, 106, 130
enzymes: digestive 1, 4–5, 61–2; supplemental 61–2; *see also* lactase
exercise 99–100

faecal microbiota transplantation (FMT) 115
fats 2, 10, 28, 32
fibre 2, 3, 34, 50–2
flatulence 8–9, 30–1, 109
FODMAPs 2, 42–7; *see also* high-FODMAP foods; low-FODMAP diet; low-FODMAP foods
food: allergens, labelling of 67–9, 73–5; allergies 39–41; and symptom diary 117–9; dairy-free 75–6, 80–1; exclusion 33; intolerance 41; intolerance testing 21; labelling 66–9; poisoning *see* gastroenteritis; *see also* 'free from' foods; elimination diet; low-FODMAP diet
'free from' foods 69–70, 132–4
fructans (FOS) 46–7, 56, 73
fructose 9, 45, 61
fruit 28, 44

galactans (GOS) 46–7, 62
GAPS diet 64
garlic 44, 45, 47, 52, 54, 71, 82
gastroenteritis xiii, 9, 19, 22, 46, 115
gluten 14, 57, 62, 73; *see also* coeliac disease; non-coeliac gluten sensitivity (NCGS)
gluten-free diet 57–8, 84; shopping for 73–5, 80–1; *see also* 'free from' foods

H. pylori 8, 19, 26
healthy eating 27–37
heartburn 8, 19, 101, 102; *see also* acid reflux
high-FODMAP foods 21, 43–5
hypnotherapy 98, 131